Managing Gout in Primary Care

Managing Gout in Primary Care

Editors
Fernando Perez-Ruiz, MD, PhD
Rheumatology Division,
Cruces University Hospital and BioCruces Health Institute.
Ana-María Herrero-Beites, MD
Physical Medicine Division,
Górliz Hospital and BioCruces Health Institute.

Contributors
Alberto Alonso-Ruiz, MD, PhD
Rheumatology Division, Cruces University Hospital and BioCruces Health Institute.
Joana Atxotegi, MD
Rheumatology Division, Cruces University Hospital and BioCruces Health Institute.
Edwin Castillo, MD
Rheumatology Division, Cruces University Hospital.
Elena Garmendia, MD, PhD
Rheumatology Division, Cruces University Hospital and BioCruces Health Institute.
Ana-María Herrero-Beites, MD
Physical Medicine Division, Górliz Hospital and BioCruces Health Institute.
Fernando Perez-Ruiz, MD, PhD
Rheumatology Division, Cruces University Hospital and BioCruces Health Institute.

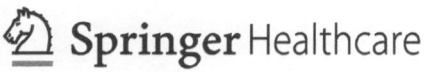

Springer Healthcare

Published by Springer Healthcare Ltd, 236 Gray's Inn Road, London, WC1X 8HB, UK.

www.springerhealthcare.com

© 2014 Springer Healthcare, a part of Springer Science+Business Media.

British Library Cataloguing-in-Publication Data.

A catalogue record for this book is available from the British Library.

ISBN 978-1-907673-66-5

Although every effort has been made to ensure that drug doses and other information are presented accurately in this publication, the ultimate responsibility rests with the prescribing physician. Neither the publisher nor the authors can be held responsible for errors or for any consequences arising from the use of the information contained herein. Any product mentioned in this publication should be used in accordance with the prescribing information prepared by the manufacturers. No claims or endorsements are made for any drug or compound at present under clinical investigation.

Project editor: Clare Shepherd
Designer: Joe Harvey
Artworker: Sissan Mollerfors
Production: Marina Maher
Printed in Great Britain by Latimer Trend

Contents

Author biographies

Fernando Perez-Ruiz (MD, PhD) gained his MD qualification in The Basque Country University in 1985. After passing the Fellowship National Examination Trial, he applied for fellowship at Hospital Ramon y Cajal in Madrid, and joined the Rheumatology Board in 1991. He is a Senior Specialist in the Rheumatology Division at Cruces University Hospital, Baracaldo, Vizcaya, Spain, where he has worked from 1991 to date as a general rheumatologist. Although initially involved with clinical investigation and publications in lupus, rheumatoid arthritis, and fibromyalgia, in the last 20 years he has focused in, and is devoted to, crystal-induced arthritis, and especially gout. He gained his PhD qualification in Barcelona University through studies of classification and urate-lowering therapy in gout. He has presented over 200 scientific communications, over 50 lectures, and published over 100 papers and book chapters, most of them involving clinical investigation in gout or pyrophosphate arthritis. Currently he is also heading the crystal-induced investigation group at the BioCruces Health Investigation Institute. He is an active member of the Spanish Society for Rheumatology (Chair of the Spanish Group for Investigation of Crystal-Induced Arthritis since 2008) and an International Member of the American College of Rheumatology. He collaborates as Associated Editor of Rheumatology International and is a member of the Editorial Committee of Bone Joint Spine, Arthritis, Seminarios de la Fundación Española de Reumatología, and Reumatología Clínica, and formerly of Arthritis Care and Research. He is also an invited reviewer for over thirty international journals. He has collaborated with the European League Against Rheumatism (EULAR) Task Force for gout, EULAR group for pyrophosphate arthritis, the Outcome Measures in Rheumatology (OMERACT) group for gout, the American College of Rheumatology (ACR) Guidelines for Gout, and has also coordinated the Spanish Guidelines for gout management.

Ana María Herrero-Beites (MD) gained her MD qualification in The Basque Country University in 1985. After passing the Fellowship National Examination Trial, she followed a fellowship program at Hospital Ramon y Cajal in Madrid from 1988, and joined the Physical Medicine Board in 1992. She is a Specialist in the Physical Medicine Division at Hospital de Górliz, Vizcaya, Spain, where she has worked from 1992 to date, initially in neurologic rehabilitation and later in musculoskeletal rehabilitation. She leads and coordinates the joint prosthesis rehabilitation process. She has closely collaborated in clinical investigation with Cruces University Hospital and is a member of the crystal-induced arthritis investigation group at BioCruces Health Institute. She has co-authored 12 papers and book chapters on musculoskeletal involvement in gout.

Alberto Alonso (MD, PhD) is a senior consultant and chief of the Rheumatology Division at Cruces University Hospital. He joined the MD board at Universidad Complutense, Madrid and the Rheumatology board after a fellowship in Ramon y Cajal Hospital in Madrid. His PhD was developed and presented in the University of the Basque Country. He serves as President of the Ethical Committee of Clinical Investigation and a member of the Corporative Commission of Pharmacy of the Health Service of the Basque Country. He has obtained three Masters Degrees of Management of Health Services, has published 82 articles and 17 book chapters and has authored over 300 papers and lectures in scientific meetings. He has been involved as the principal investigator in more than 50 clinical trials. He has also actively served as President of the Basque Society for Rheumatology, coordinator of the Postgraduate Education Committee of the Spanish Society for Rheumatology, and member of the Spanish National Specialty Committee for Rheumatology.

Joana Atxotegi (MD) is a Junior Rheumatologist at the Rheumatology Division of Cruces University Hospital. She obtained her MD at Universidad del País Vasco in 2003, and completed a fellowship in rheumatology in 2008 at the Rheumatology Division of Cruces University Hospital. She is a member of the Spanish Society of Rheumatology and has served on the Executive Committee of the Basque Country Rheumatology Society.

She has collaborated on clinical research on gout and pyrophosphate arthritis presented in national and international meetings and has authored and co-authored several papers on gout, both in national and international journals, and is principal investigator in an independent government-funded clinical trial on gout.

Edwin Castillo (MD) is the senior fellow in rheumatology at Cruces University Hospital. He obtained his MD from Universidad Industrial de Santander Medical and Health Sciences School of Colombia in 2006, and was awarded with the Rotary Graduate of Distinction. Following 4 years of medical practice, he expressed a strong interest in rheumatology and in 2010 he entered into a rheumatology fellowship in Spain. He actively collaborates with Dr Perez-Ruiz in clinical investigation in the field of crystal-induced arthritis and has co-authored publications on gout.

Elena Garmendia Sánchez (MD, PhD) is a Senior Rheumatologist at the Rheumatology Division of Cruces University Hospital. She obtained her MD at the University of the Basque Country in 1989 and completed her rheumatology training at the Rheumatology Division of Ramón y Cajal University Hospital in Madrid in 1993. She worked in the laboratory of Clinical Immunology of Medicine Department of University of Alcalá de Henares from 1994 to 1998. Her doctoral thesis was based on the study of phenotypic and functional alterations in peripheral blood lymphocytes from reactive arthritis and ankylosing spondylitis patients, obtaining a PhD degree. Her main areas of interest are within the field of spondyloarthropaties and crystal-induced arthritis, including gout and pyrophosphate arthritis, with a special focus on the role of imaging techniques. She currently combines her clinical activity with the practice of musculoskeletal ultrasound. She is a member of the Spanish Rheumatology Society, Community of Madrid Rheumatology Society and Spanish League of Rheumatology. She has served on the Executive Committee of the Basque Country Rheumatology Society and has participated in different training activities in the field of imaging, being an active member of the Ultrasound Study Group of the Spanish Society for Rheumatology.

Acknowledgments

Fernando Perez-Ruiz has been an advisor, speaker or has been involved in educational activities for Ardea Biosciences, Astra-Zeneca, Menarini, Metabolex, Novartis, Pfizer, SOBI and has received investigation funds from Ministerio de Sanidad, Gobierno de España, Sociedad Española de Reumatología, and Asociación de Reumatólogos del Hospital de Cruces.

Ana María Herrero-Beites has received investigation funds from Asociación de Reumatólogos del Hospital de Cruces.

Alberto Alonso-Ruiz has received investigation funds from Asociación de Reumatólogos del Hospital de Cruces.

Joana Atxotegi, Edwin Castillo and Elena Garmendia all declare no conflicts of interest.

Acknowledgments

Chapter 1

Disease overview

Ana María Herrero-Beites and Fernando Perez-Ruiz

Introduction

Gout has been a well-known disease for over 2000 years, and is the most common cause of joint inflammation in adult males [1]. Colchicine has been used to treat gout throughout the last three centuries [2], yet despite this, no drug was effectively and safely used to treat hyperuricemia in gout until the mid-20th century. Continued research and learning on gout slowed when allopurinol became widely available and used as a treatment option, as no unmet need was then felt to exist.

Half a century later, it became apparent that no therapeutic target based on hyperuricemia outcome had been defined. Very few controlled trials were available to test the efficacy and safety of treatments, and no research on diagnosis and management had been done despite data showing that patients with gout were generally improperly treated even in the hands of specialists [3].

In the last 10 years, good-quality evidence on gout impact and management has grown exponentially, renal transporters have been recently identified, and a number of new drugs have been approved or are under current development. The future of gout treatment therefore looks promising.

F. Perez-Ruiz and A. M. Herrero-Beites, *Managing Gout in Primary Care*,
DOI: 10.1007/978-1-907673-67-2_1, © Springer Healthcare 2014

Definitions

Hyperuricemia

Hyperuricemia can be defined in two ways. Epidemiologic and physiopathologic definitions vary, and differentiating one from another is of the utmost importance for clinical practice.

Serum urate levels differ in the population based on age and sex. As in any distribution, normality comprises the range within which 95% of the population is included. Thus, normal serum urate levels for men and women vary, the normal range being 2–7 mg/dL (120–420 μmol/L) for men and 2–6 mg/dL (120–360 μmol/L) for women, although these figures may differ between laboratories or populations. Hyperuricemia is therefore defined as serum urate levels >7 mg/dL (>420 μmol/L) for men and >6 mg/dL (>360 μmol/L) for women.

From a physiopathologic point of view, the cutoff point associated with hyperuricemia should be defined as the saturation threshold for urate under physiological conditions, which is ~6.8 mg/dL (408 μmol/L) for both men and women. This is a key concept in the understanding that the therapeutic target for urate levels in gout should be well below the saturation threshold in order to allow for spontaneous dissolution of urate crystals, as discussed in later chapters.

Gout

Gout is a deposition disease, and is therefore defined as the presence of monosodium urate crystals (MSUCs) in tissues, most commonly in articular and periarticular structures such as cartilage (Figure 1.1), tendons, and synovial membranes of joints and bursae, but also in subcutaneous tissues. These MSUCs nucleate and grow as a consequence of sustained and longstanding hyperuricemia, i.e., serum urate levels over the saturation threshold (>6.8 mg/dL [408 μmol/L]).

Tophi

A tophus is classically defined as a macroscopic subcutaneous nodule formed by deposits of MSUCs with tissue fibrous and inflammatory reactions that can be perceived on inspection or palpation during physical examination (Figure 1.2) [4].

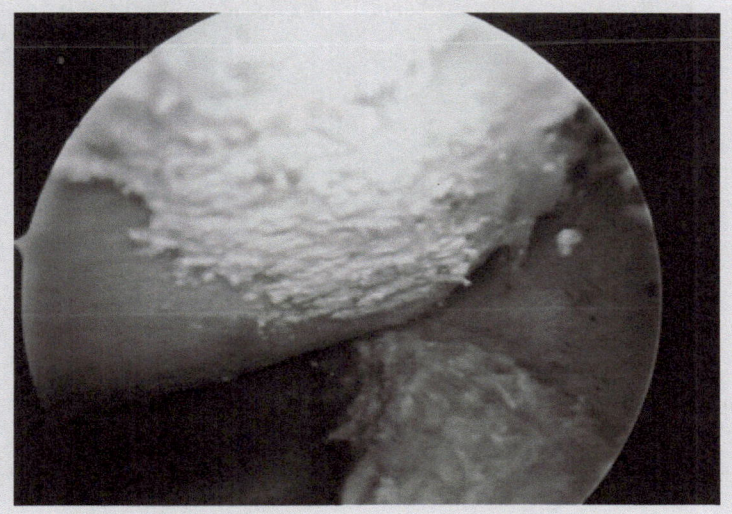

Figure 1.1 Arthroscopic image of monosodium urate crystal deposition (sugar-like cover) over the surface of the hyaline cartilage of the knee condyles. Published with kind permission of © F. Perez-Ruiz 2014. All Rights Reserved.

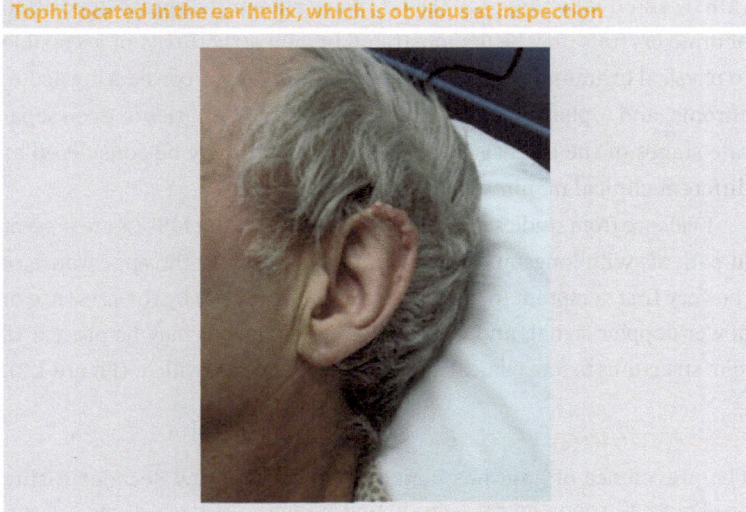

Figure 1.2 Tophi located in the ear helix, which is obvious at inspection. Published with kind permission of © F. Perez-Ruiz 2014. All Rights Reserved.

Ultrasonography of the first metatarsophalangeal joint

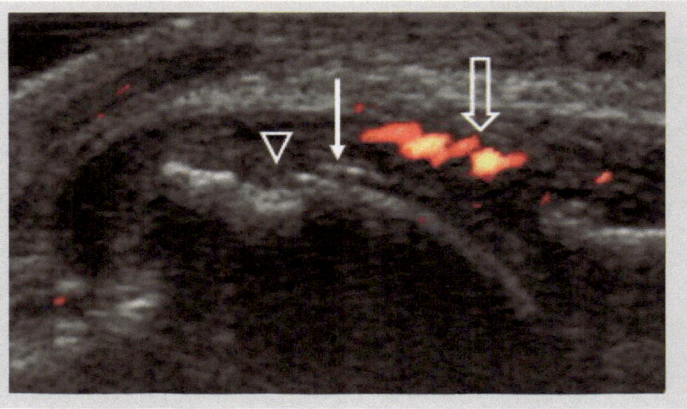

Figure 1.3 Ultrasonography of the first metatarsophalangeal joint. Showing deposition of monosodium urate crystals on the surface of the cartilage (double contour sign, arrow), nearby erosion (arrow-head), and power-doppler signal in an asymptomatic joint (open arrow). Published with kind permission of © F. Perez-Ruiz 2014. All Rights Reserved.

Nowadays, the definition of tophus needs to be considered more extensively, as new imaging techniques, such as high resolution ultrasonography (HRUS), computed tomography (CT), magnetic resonance imaging (MRI), and dual-energy CT (DECT) have shown that gross deposition of urate crystals may be demonstrated in joint structures not accessible to physical examination [5]. There is no rationale for considering acute, chronic, and tophaceous gout as different disease entities or even separate stages of the disease; instead, these may simply be considered as different clinical manifestations of gout.

Evidence from studies using HRUS demonstrate that MSUCs are present in patients with longstanding hyperuricemia prior to the appearance of the very first symptom [6,7]. Inflammation, as shown by the presence of power-doppler signal, and even subtle bone erosions may be present in joint structures before clinical manifestations become evident (Figure 1.3).

Epidemiology of gout

The prevalence of gout has increased in the last few decades, rising from 0.3% in 1990 to 0.5% in 1999 in the adult population in the US [8], with men being more commonly affected than women (4:1 in patients

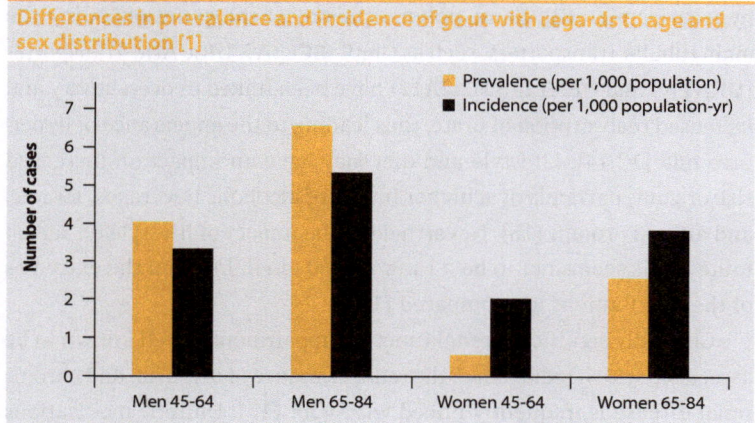

Figure 1.4 Differences in prevalence and incidence of gout with regards to age and sex distribution [1]. Published with kind permission of © F. Perez-Ruiz 2014. All Rights Reserved.

aged <65 years, 3:1 in patients >65 years) [1]. Prevalence of gout varies with age and sex, with over 6% of men and 2% of women aged >65 years suffering from gout [1].

The incidence of gout seems not to have changed in the last few decades [9]. It is also higher in men than women, and higher in the elderly population than in the younger population [1]; on average, 4–6 new cases per 1,000 population-year appear in those aged ≥65 years in a report from the UK population (Figure 1.4) [1].

Comorbidities are frequently associated with gout. About 90% of patients may show an associated comorbidity, most frequently hypertension (up to 50% of patients), hyperlipidemia (up to 60%), diabetes (up to 15%), chronic kidney disease (up to 20%), and ischemic heart disease (up to 7%) [10]. Women develop gout at an older age, are more commonly treated with diuretic medications, and show more frequent comorbidities, such as hypertension, ischemic heart disease, renal function impairment, diabetes, and peripheral artery disease, than men with gout [11].

Risk factors for hyperuricemia and gout

Hyperuricemia is the most important factor for the development of gout, and a number of diverse factors have been associated with hyperuricemia [12]. Some polymorphisms of the genes encoding the main tubular transporters, such as Glut9 (SCL2A9, URic Acid Transporter [URAT]v) and URAT1 (SCL22A12) have been linked to overactivity and increased reabsorption of urate, thus leading to the appearance of hyperuricemia [13,14]. Lifestyle and diet may have an impact on increased risk of gout, particularly a higher intake of alcoholic beverages, sweets, and animal protein [15]. Nevertheless, the impact of lifestyle on serum urate levels seems not to be >1 mg/dL (60 μmol/L) when the extremes of the distributions are compared [16].

Clinically significant renal function impairment is well known to be associated with a reduction of the renal clearance of uric acid, and chronic renal disease is frequently linked with gout [17]. Diuretic medications are the drugs that most commonly cause hyperuricemia and gout, and there is an increased risk of developing hyperuricemia and gout with the use of loop diuretics and thiazides [18].

Being overweight or obese is also a risk factor for hyperuricemia and gout [19], due to the development of insulin resistance that often occurs with these conditions [20].

Natural history of gout

Most patients with certain but untreated gout, or those not treated to target urate level to induce dissolution of MSUCs, are prone to developing a greater burden of disease. The first consequence of uncontrolled hyperuricemia in patients with gout is an increase in the number of episodes of acute inflammation (EAIs). Data from a cohort of patients seen prior to the development of urate-lowering drugs showed that the frequency of EAIs increased during follow-up in 49% of patients and severity of affliction in 29% [21]. On the contrary, sustained urate-lowering treatment to target uricemia is associated with a progressive reduction in the number of EAIs until complete resolution of symptoms [22,23]. Fewer EAIs is also associated with an improvement in perceived quality of life [24].

Another important factor is the progressive development of tophi in untreated or undertreated hyperuricemia or gout. A cohort of 392 patients with gout without previous X-ray bone erosions or osteolytic lesions, highly specific for the development of intraosseous tophi, showed a trend to lineal increase up to 47% and 70% at 10 and 20 years of follow-up, respectively (Figure 1.5) [25]. In addition, the appearance of bone lesions was dependent on the level of hyperuricemia, so that the greater the uricemia, the higher the cumulative prevalence of tophi, as shown in a cohort of 1,289 untreated patients (Figure 1.6) [26]. Conversely, treatment to target subsaturating uricemia is associated with a progressive reduction of the size of tophi [23,27], with a lower serum urate level causing more rapid reduction in tophus size, both subcutaneous [28] and articular [29].

Additionally, untreated gout can lead to the development of polyarticular joint involvement. In 178 patients with heart transplant and no previous gout, the development of high-level hyperuricemia was associated with the occurrence of gout in 22% of patients at 4-year follow-up, with 43% of that group showing polyarticular joint involvement [30]. Finally, the development of severe gout may cause structural joint damage or chronic gouty arthropathy [31], with loss of function [32] and perceived quality of life [24].

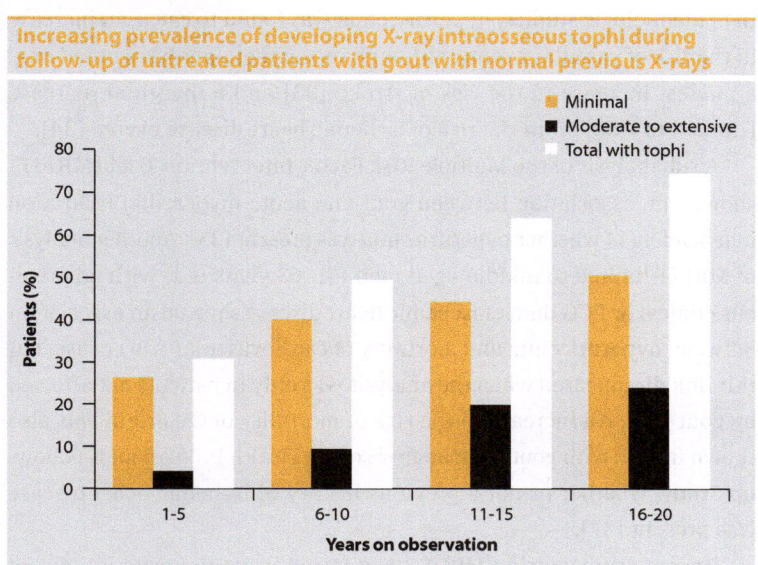

Figure 1.5 Increasing prevalence of developing X-ray intraosseous tophi during follow-up of untreated patients with gout with normal previous X-rays. Published with kind permission of © F. Perez-Ruiz 2014. All Rights Reserved.

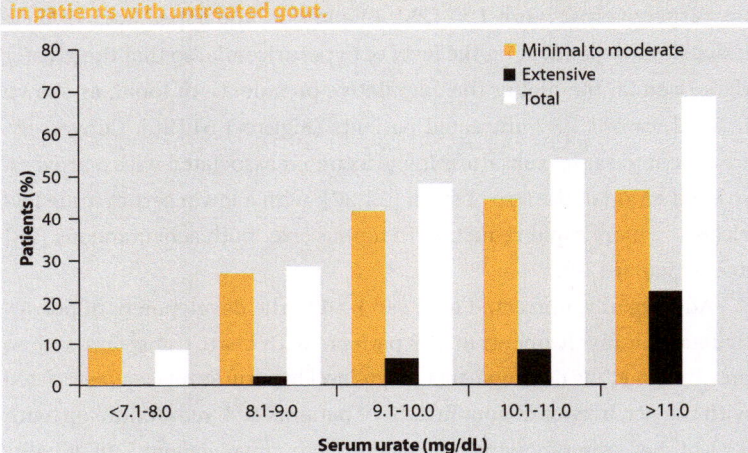

Figure 1.6 Association between serum urate levels and the risk of developing tophi in patients with untreated gout. Published with kind permission of © F. Perez-Ruiz 2014. All Rights Reserved.

Gout and vascular events

In epidemiologic studies, hyperuricemia was found to cause an increase in the risk of vascular events, although recent meta-analyses noted only a modest increase in the risk of stroke [33] and a marginal increase (limited to women) in the risk of ischemic heart disease events [34].

A subanalysis of the Multiple Risk Factor Intervention Trial (MRFIT) showed an association between gout and acute myocardial infarction independent of whether hyperuricemia was present [35]. Another analysis of MRFIT limited to middle-aged men (41–63 years old) with no previous clinical or ECG data of ischemic heart disease showed an association between hyperuricemia and mortality of cardiovascular (CV) cause, but this link disappeared when the analysis was only in patients not affected by gout [36]. An increase in the risk of mortality of CV origin was also shown in men with gout in an analysis of the Health Professionals Follow-up Study, whether or not a previous history of ischemic heart disease was present [37].

Recent studies using HRUS have found urate deposits in 34% of patients and power-doppler signal (a surrogate of inflammation) in 66% of those showing urate deposition [6].

This suggests that urate deposition precedes symptoms, and chronic inflammation is present prior to the development of the very first gout symptom. There is ultrasonographic evidence of chronic inflammation in asymptomatic joints of patients with gout, as synovial hypertrophy and moderate-to-marked power-doppler signal was observed in 68% and 28% respectively of 78 first metatarsophalangeal (MTP) joints of 39 patients, even though 22 of them were on NSAIDs [38]. The tophus represents a complex and organized chronic inflammatory tissue response to MSUCs [39], and its presence correlates with bone erosions and C-reactive protein levels [25]. In one cross-sectional study that included hyperuricemia as a confounding variable, an increasing number of affected joints was independently associated with Q-wave myocardial infarction in ECG registries in all male patients aged >50 years, and the presence of tophi was associated with the same outcome in patients aged <50 years [40]. More recently, a study based on the prospective long-term follow-up of a cohort of patients has noted that tophaceous gout is also linked to an increased risk of mortality, in most cases due to CV causes [41].

In summary, MSUC deposition, even asymptomatic and previous to any symptom, is associated with low-grade inflammation. In addition, the greater the deposition, the higher degree of chronic inflammation and the higher risk of CV complications.

The economic burden of gout

Persistence of gout symptoms is associated with loss of working days [42]. In one study, up to one in four patients aged <65 years with very frequent EAIs lost over 30 working days a year [43].

Episodes of EAIs, also known as 'flares,' 'attacks,' or 'relapses,' have also been connected to greater healthcare costs, mostly generated by repeated visits to primary care physicians, especially for patients with associated comorbidities [44]. Increased number of visits to emergency rooms and all-cause hospitalizations have also been described [45].

Although the presence of uncontrolled urate levels in patients with gout may be attributed to lack of compliance with medication [46], poor control of hyperuricemia has been demonstrated in studies even in a majority of patients treated by specialists [3]. Proper information, education, setting of targets, and adequate follow-up seem to be appropriate goals for proper control of gout [47]. In summary, gout is no longer considered to be associated with overindulgence and gluttony. A genetic predisposition is now well known, and although lifestyle factors may contribute to the development of hyperuricemia, a considerable number of patients, especially the elderly, suffer from gout secondary to medication or chronic renal disease. A well-planned approach to the diagnosis, evaluation, and treatment of gout will lead to improvements in the management of this disease [48].

Key points

- Gout is defined by the presence of MSUCs in tissues due to longstanding hyperuricemia.
- Gout is the most common inflammatory arthritis condition in adults; its prevalence is greater in the elderly due to concomitant disease and medication.
- The natural history of untreated or undertreated gout is the development of crippling, tophaceous, polyarticular joints with destructive involvement.
- Recurrent episodes, inflammation, and chronic symptoms are associated with decreased perceived quality of life and increased health and economic expenses.
- Increasing evidence is linking gout to a greater risk of CV events.

References

1   Mikuls TR, Farrar JT, Bilker WB, Fernandes S, Schumacher HR Jr, Saag KG. Gout epidemiology: results from the UK General Practice Research Database, 1990–1999. *Ann Rheum Dis*. 2005;64:267-272.
2   Terkeltaub RA. Colchicine update: 2008. Semin Arthritis Rheum. 2009;38:411-419.
3   Perez-Ruiz F, Carmona L, Yébenes MJG, et al; on behalf of the GEMA Study Group, Sociedad Española de Reumatología. An audit of the variability of diagnosis and management of gout in the rheumatology setting: the Gout Evaluation and Management study. *J Clin Rheumatol*. 2011;17:349-355.
4   Campion EW, Glynn RJ, DeLabry LO. Asymptomatic hyperuricemia. Risks and consequences in the normative aging study. *Am J Med*. 1987;82:421-426.
5   Perez-Ruiz F, Dalbeth N, Urresola A, de Miguel E, Schlesinger N. Imaging of gout: findings and utility. *Arthritis Res Ther*. 2009;11:232.

6 Puig JG, de Miguel E, Castillo MC, López Rocha A, Martínez MA, Torres RJ. Asymptomatic hyperuricemia: impact of ultrasonography. *Nucleosides Nucleotides Nucleic Acids.* 2008;27:592-595.

7 Pineda C, Amezcua-Guerra LM, Solano C, et al. Joint and tendon subclinical involvement suggestive of gouty arthritis in asymptomatic hyperuricemia: an ultrasound controlled study. *Arthritis Res Ther.* 2011;13:R4.

8 Wallace KL, Riedel AA, Joseph-Ridge N, Wortmann R. Increasing prevalence of gout and hyperuricemia over 10 years among older adults in a managed care population. *J Rheumatol.* 2004;31:1582-1587.

9 Cea Soriano L, Rothenbacher D, Choi HK, García Rodríguez LA. Contemporary epidemiology of gout in the UK general population. *Arthritis Res Ther.* 2011;13:R39.

10 Smith EUR, Díaz-Torné C, Perez-Ruiz F, March LM. Epidemiology of gout: an update. *Best Pract Res Clin Rheumatol.* 2010;24:811-827.

11 Harrold LR, Yood RA, Mikuls TR, et al. Sex differences in gout epidemiology: evaluation and treatment. *Ann Rheum Dis.* 2006;65:1368-1372.

12 Singh JA, Reddy SG, Kundukulam J. Risk factors for gout and prevention: a systematic review of the literature. *Curr Opin Rheumatol.* 2011;23:192-202.

13 Enomoto A, Endou H. Roles of organic anion transporters (OATs) and a urate transporter (URAT1) in the pathophysiology of human disease. *Clin Exp Nephrol.* 2005;9:195-205.

14 Anzai N, Ichida K, Jutabha P, et al. Plasma urate level is directly regulated by a voltage-driven urate efflux transporter URATv1 (*SLC2A9*) in humans. *J Biol Chem.* 2008;283:26834-26838.

15 Choi HK, Curhan G. Gout: epidemiology and lifestyle choices. *Curr Opin Rheumatol.* 2005;17:341-345.

16 Perez Ruiz F, Herrero-Beites AM. Evaluation and treatment of gout as a chronic disease. *Adv Ther.* 2012;29:935-946.

17 Avram Z, Krishnan E. Hyperuricemia—where nephrology meets rheumatology. *Rheumatology (Oxford).* 2010;47:960-964.

18 McAdams DeMarco MA, Maynard JW, Baer AN, et al. Diuretic use, increased serum urate and the risk of incident gout in a population-based study of hypertensive adults: the Atherosclerosis Risk in the Communities cohort. *Arthritis Rheum.* 2012;64:121-129.

19 Choi HK, Atkinson K, Karlson EW, Curhan G. Obesity, weight change, hypertension, diuretic use, and risk of gout in men: the health professionals follow-up study. *Arch Intern Med.* 2005;165:742-748.

20 Choi HK, Ford ES. Haemoglobin A1c, fasting glucose, serum C-peptide and insulin resistance in relation to serum uric acid levels—the Third National Health and Nutrition Examination Survey. *Rheumatology (Oxford).* 2008;47:713-717.

21 Gutman AB. Treatment of primary gout: the present status. Arthitis Rheum. 1965;8:911-920.

22 Perez-Ruiz F, Calabozo M, Fernandez-Lopez MJ, et al. Treatment of chronic gout in patients with renal function impairment: an open, randomized, actively controlled study. *J Clin Rheumatol.* 1999;5:49-55.

23 Becker MA, Schumacher HR, MacDonald PA, Lloyd E, Lademacher C. Clinical efficacy and safety of successful longterm urate lowering with febuxostat or allopurinol in subjects with gout. *J Rheumatol.* 2009;36:1273-1282.

24 Khanna PP, Perez-Ruiz F, Maranian P, Khanna D. Long-term therapy for chronic gout results in clinically important improvements in the health-related quality of life: short form-36 is responsive to change in chronic gout. *Rheumatology (Oxford).* 2011;50:740-745.

25 Dalbeth N, Clark B, Gregory K, et al. Mechanisms of bone erosions in gout: a quantitative analysis using plain radiography and computed tomography. *Ann Rheum Dis.* 2009;68:1290-1295.

26 Gutman AB. The past four decades of progress in the knowledge of gout, with an assessment of the present status. *Arthritis Rheum.* 1973;16:431-445.

27 Schumacher HR Jr, Becker MA, Lloyd E, MacDonald PA, Lademacher C. Febuxostat in the treatment of gout: 5-yr findings of the FOCUS efficacy and safety study. *Rheumatology (Oxford).* 2009;48:188-194.

28 Perez-Ruiz F, Calabozo M, Pijoan JI, Herrero-Beites AM, Ruibal A. Effect of urate-lowering therapy on the velocity of size reduction of tophi in chronic gout. *Arthritis Rheum.* 2002;47:356-360.

29 Perez-Ruiz F, Martin I, Canteli B. Ultrasonographic measurement of tophi as an outcome measure for chronic gout. *J Rheumatol.* 2007;34:1888-1893.

30 Burack DA, Griffith BP, Thompson ME, Kahl LE. Hyperuricemia and gout among heart transplant patients receiving cyclosporine. *Am J Med.* 1992;92:141-146.

31 Dalbeth N, Clark B, McQueen F, Doyle A, Taylor W. Validation of a radiographic damage index in chronic gout. *Arthritis Rheum.* 2007;57:1067-1073.

32 Dalbeth N, Collis J, Gregory K, Clark B, Robinson E, McQueen FM. Tophaceous joint disease strongly predicts hand function in patients with gout. Rheumatology. 2007;46:1804-1807.

33 Kim SY, Guevara JP, Kim KM, Choi HK, Heitjan DF, Albert DA. Hyperuricemia and risk of stroke: a systematic review and meta-analysis. *Arthritis Rheum.* 2009;61:885-892.

34 Kim SY, Guevara JP, Kim KM, Choi HK, Heitjan DF, Albert DA. Hyperuricemia and coronary heart disease: a systematic review and meta-analysis. *Arthitis Care Res (Hoboken).* 2010;62:170-180.

35 Krishnan E, Baker JF, Furst DE, Schumacher HR. Gout and the risk of acute myocardial infarction. *Arthritis Rheum.* 2006;54:2688-2696.

36 Krishnan E, Svendsen K, Neaton JD, Grandits G, Kuller LH; MRFIT Research Group. Long-term cardiovascular mortality among middle-aged men with gout. *Arch Intern Med.* 2008;168: 1104-1110.

37 Choi HK, Curhan G. Independent impact of gout on mortality and risk for coronary heart disease. *Circulation.* 2007;116:894-900.

38 Wright SA, Filippucci E, McVeigh C, et al. High resolution ultrasonography of the first metatarsal phalangeal joint in gout: a controlled study. *Ann Rheum Dis.* 2007;66:859-864.

39 Dalbeth N, Pool B, Gamble G, et al. Cellular characterization of the gouty tophus: a quantitative analysis [abstract]. *Arthitis Rheum.* 2009;60(suppl 10):1948.

40 Chen SY, Chen CL, Shen ML. Severity of gouty arthritis is associated with Q-wave myocardial infarction: a large-scale, cross-sectional study. *Clin Rheumatol.* 2007;26:308-313.

41 Perez-Ruiz F, Martinez-Indart L, Carmona L, Herrero-Beites AM, Pijoan JI, Krishnan E. Tophaceous gout and high level of hyperuricaemia are both associated with increased risk of mortality in patients with gout [published online ahead of print January 12, 2013]. *Ann Rheum Dis.* doi:10.1136/annrheumdis-2012-202421.

42 Lynch W, Chan W, Kleinman N, Andrews LM, Yadao AM. Economic burden of gouty arthritis attacks for employees with frequent and infrequent attacks. *Popul Health Manag.* 2013:16; 138-145.

43 Edwards NL, Sundy JS, Forsythe A, Blume S, Pan F, Becker MA. Work productivity loss dueto flares in patients with chronic gout refractory to conventional therapy. *J Med Econ.* 2011;14: 10-15.

44 Sicras-Mainar A, Navarro-Artieda R, Ibáñez-Nolla J. Resource use and economic impact of patients with gout: a multicenter, population-wide study. *Reumatol Clin.* 2013;9:94-100.

45 Park H, Rascati KL, Prasla K, McBayne T. Evaluation of health care costs and utilization patterns for patients with gout. *Clin Ther.* 2012;34:640-652.

46 Riedel AA, Nelson M, Joseph-Ridge N, Wallace K, MacDonald PA, Becker M. Compliance with allopurinol therapy among managed care enrollees with gout: a retrospective analysis of administrative claims. *J Rheumatol.* 2004;31:1575-1581.

47 Rees F, Jenkins W, Doherty M. Patients with gout adhere to curative treatment if informed appropriately: proof-of-concept observational study. Ann Rheum Dis. 2013;72:826-830.

48 Doherty M, Jansen TL, Nuki G, et al. Gout: why is this curable disease so seldom cured? *Ann Rheum Dis.* 2012;71:1765-1770.

Chapter 2

Physiopathology of gout

Fernando Perez-Ruiz and Edwin Castillo

Introduction

Gout can be defined as the presence of monosodium urate crystals (MSUCs) in tissues. These MSUCs may induce acute inflammation when shed into the synovial fluid or cause aggregate-inducing chronic tissue inflammation.

The nucleation and formation of MSUCs is related to the presence of longstanding hyperuricemia, which is an essential factor in the development of gout. Other factors, such as level of hyperuricemia, time exposed to hyperuricemia, and genetic or acquired tissue predisposition for the nucleation of MSUCs, may explain why not all patients with hyperuricemia develop gout, or why some patients develop early or rapidly progressive symptoms associated with gout.

Genetic factors associated with hyperuricemia

The organic anion transporter family, located primarily in the proximal renal tubules, is responsible for most of the renal handling of uric acid. Multiple renal tubular transporters have been identified, but the most important ones seem to be uric acid transporter (URAT)1 [1] and URAT1v [2], with their lack of expression leading to renal hypouricemia types 1 and 2, respectively. Polymorphisms encoding hyperactive variants of these renal tubular transporters have been associated with increased risk of hyperuricemia and gout [3]. More recently, a new transporter, ABCG2 has emerged as a major contributor to impaired intestinal excretion of uric acid [4].

F. Perez-Ruiz and A. M. Herrero-Beites, *Managing Gout in Primary Care*,   13
DOI: 10.1007/978-1-907673-67-2_2, © Springer Healthcare 2014

URAT1 is the product of the *SCL22A12* gene. It is expressed only in the kidney and is located in the epithelium of the proximal (but not the distal) renal tubules at the apical membrane (luminal side). URAT1-deficient mice and humans show complete loss of the capacity to reabsorb uric acid, with correspondingly extremely low serum urate (sUr) levels and increased risk of renal lithiasis [5]. The majority of the drugs known to exert a significant uricosuric effect share the ability to inhibit URAT1. In contrast, most diuretic medications that induce a rise in sUr also increase uric acid URAT1-mediated transport [5]. The most effective uricosuric drug tested in clinical practice is benzbromarone, a drug that exerts intense inhibition of URAT1 activity, although is not widely available for clinical use [6].

The facilitated glucose transporter Glut9 was also found to act as a voltage-driven urate transporter and is therefore also known as URATv1 (voltage-driven urate transporter 1) [2]. Located mainly in the kidney and in the liver, Glut9 is encoded by the *SCL2A9* gene and is present both in the apical and basolateral membranes of the proximal tubule epithelial cells [2]. It shows different substrate affinities compared with URAT1; it is not influenced by organic anions, and hexoses strongly inhibit uric acid transport via Glut9. There are two known variants or isoforms of Glut9 (long and short, or Glut9a and Glut 9b), each showing different functionality depending on the intracellular concentration of hexoses [7]. Functional cooperation between URAT1 and URATv1 may be needed for maintaining uric acid homeostasis at the renal level [8].

Recent genome-wide association studies of sUr have identified an adenosine triphosphate-binding cassette transporter from sub-family G, member 2 (ABCG2). It is a unidirectional transporter located in the renal tubule and intestines, and its lack of expression has been associated with decreased intestinal excretion of uric acid [9].

Because urate deposition is enhanced in joints with osteoarthritis or cartilage derangements, it has been suggested that genetic factors related to matrix glycoproteins may also influence the deposition of urate crystals acting as templates for nucleation [10].

Mechanisms of hyperuricemia

Hyperuricemia is uncommon in animals. Humans and upper apes show higher serum urate levels than other mammals due to the loss of expression of the gene encoding uricase [11], which cleaves uric acid to allantoin, a more water soluble purine end-product. Renal excretion makes up about two-thirds of uric acid excretion; intestinal excretion may comprise up to one-third of that in people with normal renal function (defined in Chapter 1), and may even increase in patients with impaired renal function.

Several mechanisms, either alone or in combination, may explain why sUr rises over the concentration expected for those with normal function: an increase in the production of uric acid and inefficient renal excretion (IRE) and intestinal excretion of uric acid (Figure 2.1).

Inefficient renal excretion of uric acid ('renal underexcretion')

Up to 90% of patients with gout show IRE of uric acid [12]. It is clinically and academically attractive to differentiate patients who have IRE of uric acid, as it may help to better understand the underlying mechanisms and facilitate differential diagnosis. As we can only ascertain the presence of IRE of uric acid, those patients showing efficient renal excretion will be classified as having increased production or decreased intestinal excretion (or 'false overproduction,' as shown later).

Different methods have been proposed to identify patients with gout who have IRE of uric acid: 24-hour urinary uric acid (24-Uur) excretion [13]; clearance of uric acid (CuA) [12]; the urine uric acid-to-creatinine ratio [14]; the uric acid excretion per glomerular filtration volume, or Simkin's Index [15]; and fractional excretion of uric acid. Some investigators have even suggested a composite method to simplify this assessment [16]. The first two methods require 24-hour urine collection, whilst the latter three may be calculated using spot urine and blood samples.

Renal clearance gives an indication of the renal capacity to clear blood of any solute. Clearance of uric acid shows a good correlation with 24-Uur and fractional excretion in patients with normal renal function [17], but cumbersome 12- to 24-hour urine collections are needed to measure it.

Mechanisms and causes of longstanding hyperuricemia leading to gout

1. Primary

a. Increased production of uric acid (<10%)

Idiopathic

Phosphofructokinase deficiency

Hypoxanthine-guanine-phosphoribosyl transferase deficiency

    Partial (Seegmiller-Kelley Syndrome)

    Complete (Lesch-Nyhan Syndrome)

Phosphoribosyl-pyrophosphate-synthetase overactivity

Glucogenosis (I, III, V and VII)

b. Inefficient excretion (>90%)

Idiopathic (transporter overactivity)

Familial juvenile nephropathy with hyperuricemia (uromoduline mutation)

2. Acquired

a. Increased production

Exogenous (diet related)

Ethanol

Purines and animal proteins

Increased cellular turnover

Extensive psoriasis

Chronic myeloid/lymphoid proliferative diseases

Chronic corpustular hemolythic anemia

b. Inefficient excretion

Medications

Diuretics (high-dose thiazides)

Transplant agents (cyclosporine A, tacrolimus)

Salicylic acid, phenylbutazone (low dose)

Antibiotics (pyrazinamide, ethambutol)

Anti-HIV agents (didanosine, ritonavir)

Diet related

Sweetened (fructose-rich) food and drink

Hypercaloric diet (insulin resistance)

c. Renal diseases

Arterial hypertension

Chronic renal disease

Figure 2.1 Mechanisms and causes of longstanding hyperuricemia leading to gout.
Published with kind permission of © F. Perez-Ruiz 2014. All Rights Reserved.

Fractional excretion is an inexpensive method that uses spot blood and urine samples, and has been found to correlate with clearance in patients with normal renal function [18]. Only fractional excretion and clearance remain unchanged in patients treated with xanthine oxidase inhibitors (XOI)[12] and may be used to estimate IRE of uric acid in patients with ongoing XOI use. A limitation to the use of fractional excretion is that it is not useful in patients with decreased glomerular filtration rate [17].

Increase in uric acid production ('overproduction')

An increase in uric acid production may be due to several different mechanisms. It is generally assumed that this increase comprises 5–10% of all causes of hyperuricemia [12].

One mechanism of overproduction is through genetic alterations that lead to defects in the enzymes responsible for uric acid metabolism, leading to an increase in endogenous uric acid production. These kinds of anomalies, such as in Lesch-Nyhan Syndrome or glycogen storage disease type I (von Gierke's disease) and V (McArdle disease), among others, are rare enzyme deficiencies. A second mechanism is the increase in cellular turnover that may be seen in several different corpuscular anemia or lymphoid or myeloid proliferative conditions [19]. Another is excessive exogenous supply of purines due to a diet rich in high purine-containing food [20]. There is no way to ascertain a mechanism of overproduction, although genetic testing can be carried out when there is a definite suspicion of a genetic cause.

Impaired intestinal excretion

Recently, Ichida et al. showed that decreased activity of the ABCG2 transporter was associated with decreased intestinal excretion of uric acid and renal overload, or 'false overproduction' [4]. Therefore, patients with normal renal function and efficient renal excretion may have either increased production of uric acid or decreased intestinal excretion of uric acid.

Until genetic tests for these transporters become inexpensive and widespread for clinical practice, evaluation of renal excretion of uric acid (fractional excretion for patients with normal renal function and clearance of uric acid for patients with chronic kidney disease) will remain the only clinical clue to the mechanism causing hyperuricemia.

Mechanisms of inflammation and joint damage in gout

The deposition of MSUCs in the joints seems to first appear in the surface of the hyaline cartilage. There is a shedding of crystals to the synovial fluid that may sensitize resident monocytes into active pro-inflammatory macrophages that would react when primed with new fresh crystals (Figure 2.2) [21]. There appears to be a threshold to induce acute, symptomatic inflammation, as chronic subclinical inflammation has been found in synovial fluid of asymptomatic joints showing persistence of MSUCs [22], and there is a presence of power-doppler signal in patients showing MSUC deposition by ultrasonography [23] (see Chapter 3 for imaging).

The NALP3 inflammasome has been recently considered to be one of the major routes of crystal-induced inflammation. The inflammasome is a protein complex component of innate immunity; activation of NALP3 induces activation of caspase 1 that cleaves pro-interleukin 1 into interleukin-1β (IL-1β). Interleukin-1β interacts with its receptor (which is dependent on toll-like receptors), activating a myeloid-differentiation protein (MyD88) that induces nuclear factor-kappa B and thus the release of several pro-inflammatory cytokines, metalloproteases, and radical

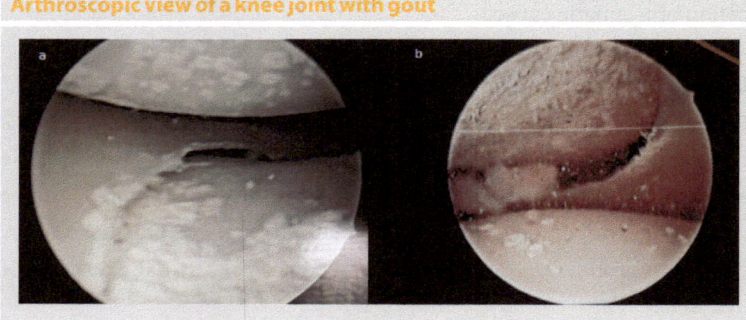

Arthroscopic view of a knee joint with gout

Figure 2.2 Arthroscopic view of a knee joint with gout. Deposition of MSUCs is initiated in the surface of hyaline cartilage (a). Crystals may shed into the synovial fluid (b) due to mechanical stress or changes in physiochemical conditions. Published with kind permission of © F. Perez-Ruiz 2014. All Rights Reserved.

oxygen species (ROS) [24]. The final result is an intense recruitment of neutrophil leukocytes that can be observed in synovial fluid heavily infiltrating the synovial membrane (Figure 2.3) [25].

An increase of MSUC deposition in the cartilage surface and consistent shedding into the synovial fluid will lead to their deposition in the synovial membrane, resulting in chronic granulomatous 'foreign-body'

Synovial fluid and synovial membrane findings during the acute episodes of inflammation

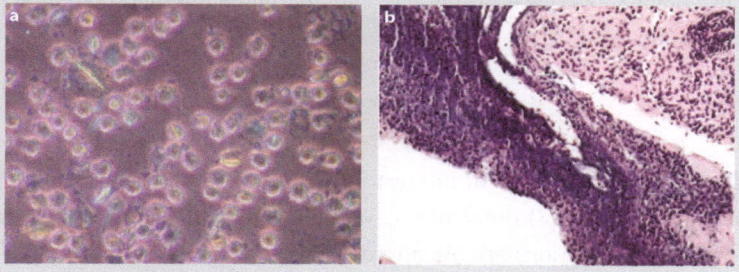

Figure 2.3 Synovial fluid and synovial membrane findings during the acute episodes of inflammation. The load of crystals into the synovial space may trigger phagocytosis by phagocytes (a: synovial fluid sample; polarized, contrast-phase microscopy, 400x), activate different cascades of inflammatory responses, and induce further recruitment through acute neutrophylic infiltration of the synovial membrane (b: synovial membrane biopsy, hematoxylin-eosine). Published with kind permission of © F. Perez-Ruiz 2014. All Rights Reserved.

Chronic urate-induced granulomatous synovitis

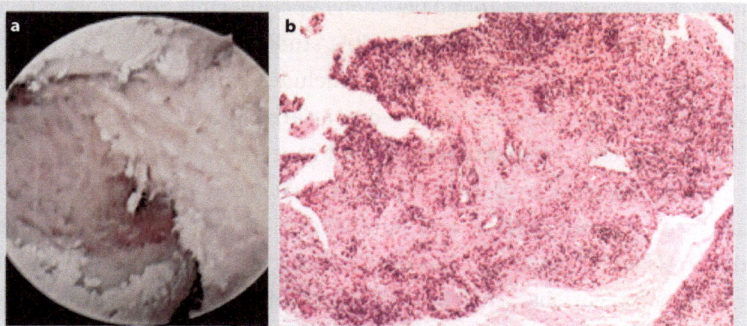

Figure 2.4 Chronic urate-induced granulomatous synovitis. Persistence of MSUCs in untreated or undertreated gout induces chronic synovial membrane inflammation (a: arthroscopic view), with chronic granulomatous 'foreign-body'-like inflammatory reaction (b: synovial membrane biopsy showing epithelial palisades and multinucleated cells, hematoxylin-eosine). Published with kind permission of © F. Perez-Ruiz 2014. All Rights Reserved.

inflammation (Figure 2.4). The granulomatous reaction to the deposition of MSUCs has been studied in tophaceous deposition, showing that a large number of cells express IL-1β [26]. Therefore, IL-1 seems to be a mediator of both acute and chronic inflammation, which makes IL-1 blockade a promising therapeutic target in gout [27] (see Chapter 5).

The development of MSUC deposition associated with chronic inflammation within the joint, or intra-articular tophi that may not be perceived in clinical examination [28], seems to be the mechanism for the development of bone erosions and, later, permanent structural damage of the joint [29].

Chronic inflammation in gout and its association with cardiovascular outcomes

Currently, there is a great interest in the impact of hyperuricemia on cardiovascular (CV) outcomes; nevertheless, in most countries urate lowering medications are not approved for the treatment of asymptomatic hyperuricemia.

The impact of hyperuricemia on CV events has been shown to be mild-to-moderate in recent systematic reviews and meta-analyses [30,31]. A meta-analysis that included 26 studies of over 400,000 adults only found a significant association between hyperuricemia and coronary heart disease (CHD) incidence or mortality in women, not in men [30]. A modest association was found between hyperuricemia and stroke when over 200,000 patients from 16 eligible studies were pooled for meta-analysis [31]. In none of the studies included in either meta-analysis was the presence of gout considered as a variable, so it is not known for certain how many patients actually had gout [32].

When 'presence or absence of gout' is available as a variable for analysis, a certain independent and significant association between a gout diagnosis and CV outcomes has been noted, even when other associated confounding variables such as CHD, heart failure, and myocardial dysfunction have been included [33–35]. Put simply, the difference between hyperuricemia and gout is that gout is a condition in which deposition of MSUCs in tissue has occurred, eliciting acute, chronic, and even subclinical inflammation.

Asymptomatic longstanding hyperuricemia is associated with urate deposition and subclinical inflammation previous to clinical gout development. In patients with longstanding asymptomatic hyperuricemia, urate deposits were observed in 34% and power-doppler signal was present in 66% [23].

Subclinical inflammation is present in asymptomatic joints of patients with gout [22]. Ultrasonographic evidence has supported this, as synovial hypertrophy and moderate-to-marked power-doppler signal was observed in 68% and 28%, retrospectively, of 78 first MTP joints of 39 patients, despite the fact that 22 of them were on NSAIDs [36].

Extensive MSUC deposition is associated with chronic histopathologic inflammation, elevated C-reactive protein, and CV outcomes. As previously mentioned, tophi represent a complex and organized chronic inflammatory tissue response to MSUCs [26]. It is agreed that the highest burden of MSUC deposition is the chronic inflammatory response, so the question that remains is to ascertain whether severity of gout, as a hallmark of the burden of deposition, is associated with CV outcomes.

In one cross-sectional study that included hyperuricemia as a confounding variable, an increased number of affected joints was independently associated with Q-wave myocardial infarction in electrocardiogram registries in all patients (men aged >50 years) and the presence of tophi was associated with the same outcome in patients aged <50 years [37]. More recently, a study based on the prospective long-term follow-up of a cohort of patients has shown that tophaceous gout is also associated with increased risk of mortality, in most cases due to CV origin [38].

Treatment of gout with colchicine decreases MSUC-induced inflammation and CV events. Colchicine therapy has been shown to reduce leukocyte counts in synovial fluids of asymptomatic joints containing MSUCs [39]. In a recent cross-sectional, retrospective study of over 12,000 patients, those who had ever been treated with colchicine had a lower rate of myocardial infarction that persisted whether or not allopurinol intake was considered as a confounding variable [40]. Patients treated with colchicine also exhibited trends toward reduced all-cause mortality and lower C-reactive protein levels [40].

Key points

- Prolonged hyperuricemia is the fundamental contributing factor to MSUC formation.
- Both genetic and environmental factors contribute to the development of hyperuricemia, and therefore of gout. Local tissue factors may also be a factor in MSUC nucleation and growth.
- Persistence of MSUCs may trigger both acute inflammatory responses and chronic inflammation responsible for the later destruction of osteoarticular structures.
- Recent data show an association between chronic urate deposition and CV events that may occur through the persistence of chronic subclinical inflammation.
- A greater burden of deposition may be linked to poorer CV outcomes.

References

1 Enomoto A, Kimura H, Chairoungdua A, et al. Molecular identification of a renal urate–anion exchanger that regulates blood urate levels. *Nature*. 2002;417:447-452.

2 Anzai N, Ichida K, Jutabha P, et al. Plasma urate level is directly regulated by a voltage-driven urate efflux transporter URATv1 (*SLC2A9*) in humans. *J Biol Chem*. 2008;283:26834-26838.

3 Kolz M, Johnson T, Sanna S, et al. Meta-analysis of 28,141 individuals identifies common variants within five new loci that influence uric acid concentrations. *PLoS Genet*. 2009;5:e1000504.

4 Ichida K, Matsuo H, Takada T, et al. Decreased extra-renal urate excretion is a common cause of hyperuricemia. *Nat Commun*. 2012;3:764.

5 Enomoto A, Endou H. Roles of organic anion transporters (OATs) and a urate transporter (URAT1) in the pathophysiology of human disease. *Clin Exp Nephrol*. 2005;9:195-205.

6 Perez-Ruiz F, Alonso-Ruiz A, Calabozo M, Herrero-Beites A, Garcia-Erauskin G, Ruiz-Lucea E. Efficacy of allopurinol and benzbromarone for the control of hyperuricaemia. A pathogenic approach to the treatment of primary chronic gout. *Ann Rheum Dis*. 1998;57:545-549.

7 Witkowska K, Smith KM, Yao SYM, et al. Human SLC2A9a and SLC2A9b isoforms mediate electrogenic transport of urate with different characteristics in the presence of hexoses. *Am J Physiol Renal Physiol*. 2012;303:F527-F539.

8 Nakanishi T, Ohya K, Shimada S, Anzai N, Tamai I. Functional cooperation of URAT1 (*SLC22A12*) and URATv1 (*SLC2A9*) in renal reabsorption of urate. *Nephrol Dial Transplant*. 2013;28:603-611.

9 Matsuo H, Takada T, Ichida K, et al. Common defects of ABCG2, a high-capacity urate exporter, cause gout: a function-based genetic analysis in a Japanese population. *Sci Transl Med*. 2009;1:5ra11.

10 Pascual E, Martínez A, Ordóñez S. Gout: the mechanism of urate crystal nucleation and growth. A hypothesis based in facts. *Joint Bone Spine*. 2013;80:1-4.

11 Johnson RJ, Andrews P, Benner SA, Oliver W. Theodore E. Woodward Award: The evolution of obesity: insights from the mid-Miocene. *Trans Am Clin Climat Assoc*. 2010;121:295-308.

12 Wortmann RL, Fox IH. Limited value of uric acid to creatinine ratios in estimating uric acid excretion. *Ann Intern Med*. 1980;93:822-825.

13 Perez-Ruiz F, Calabozo M, García Erauskin G, Ruibal A, Herrero-Beites AM. Renal underexcretion of uric acid is present in patients with apparent high urinary uric acid output. *Arthritis Rheum*. 2002;47:610-613.

14 Moriwaki Y, Yamamoto T, Takahashi S, Yamakita J, Tsutsumi Z, Hada T. Spot urine uric acid to creatinine ratio used in the estimation of uric acid excretion in primary gout. *J Rheumatol*. 2001;28:1306-1310.

15 Simkin PA, Hoover PL, Paxson CS, Wilson WF. Uric acid excretion: quantitative assessment from spot, midmorning serum and urine samples. *Ann Intern Med*. 1979;91:44-47.

16 Yamamoto T, Moriwaki Y, Takahashi S, et al. A simple method of selecting gout patients for treatment with uricosuric agents, using spot urine and blood samples. *J Rheumatol*. 2002;29:1937-1941.

17 Perez-Ruiz F, Herrero-Beites AM. Reply to letter: new standards for uric acid excretion and evidence for an inducible transporter. *Arthritis Care Res*. 2003;49:736-737.

18 Kannangara DRW, Ramasamy SN, Indraratna PL, et al. Fractional clearance of urate: validation of measurement in spot-urine samples in healthy subjects and gouty patients. *Arthritis Res Ther*. 2012;14:R189.

19 Gutman AB, Yü TF. Gout, a derangement of purine metabolism. *Adv Inter Med*. 1952;7:227-302.

20 Choi HK, Liu S, Curhan G. Intake of purine-rich foods, protein, and dairy products and relationship to serum levels of uric acid: the Third National Health and Nutrition Examination Survey. *Arthritis Rheum*. 2005;52:283-289.

21 Martin WJ, Shaw O, Liu X, Steiger S, Harper JL. Monosodium urate monohydrate crystal–recruited non-inflammatory monocytes differentiate into M1-like pro-inflammatory macrophages in a peritoneal murine model of gout. *Arthritis Rheum*. 2011;63:1322-1332.

22 Pascual E. Persistence of monosodium urate crystals and low-grade inflammation in synovial fluid of patients with untreated gout. *Arthritis Rheum*. 1991;34:141-145.

23 Puig JG, de Miguel E, Castillo MC, López Rocha A, Martínez MA, Torres RJ. Asymptomatic hyperuricemia: impact of ultrasonography. *Nucleosides Nucleotides Nucleic Acids*. 2008;27: 592-595.

24 Reginato AM, Olsen BR. Genetics and experimental models of crystal-induced arthritis. Lessons learned from mice and men: is it crystal clear? Curr Opin Rheumatol. 2009;19:134-145.

25 Schumacher HR. Pathology of the synovial membrane in gout. Light and electron microscopic studies. *Arthritis Rheum*. 1975;18:771-782.

26 Dalbeth N, Pool B, Gamble G, et al. Cellular characterization of the gouty tophus: a quantitative analysis [abstract]. *Arthitis Rheum*. 2009;60(suppl 10:1948.

27 So A, Busso N. A magic bullet for gout? *Ann Rheum Dis*. 2009;68:1517-1519.

28 Perez-Ruiz F, Martin I, Canteli B. Ultrasonographic measurement of tophi as an outcome measure for chronic gout. *J Rheumatol*. 2007;34:1888-1893.

29 Dalbeth N, Clark B, Gregory K, et al. Mechanisms of bone erosions in gout: a quantitative analysis using plain radiography and computed tomography. *Ann Rheum Dis*. 2009;68: 1290-1295.

30 Kim SY, Guevara JP, Kim KM, Choi HK, Heitjan DF, Albert DA. Hyperuricemia and coronary heart disease: a systematic review and meta-analysis. Arthitis Care Res (Hoboken). 2010;62:170-180.

31 Kim SY, Guevara JP, Kim KM, Choi HK, Heitjan DF, Albert DA. Hyperuricemia and risk of stroke: a systematic review and meta-analysis. *Arthritis Rheum*. 2009;61:885-892.

32 Zhu Y, Pandya BJ, Choi HK. Prevalence of gout and hyperuricemia in the US general population: the National Health and Nutrition Examination Survey 2007–2008. *Arthritis Rheum*. 2011;63:3136-3141.

33 Krishnan E, Baker JF, Furst DE, Schumacher HR. Gout and the risk of acute myocardial infarction. *Arthritis Rheum*. 2006;54:2688-2696.

34 Krishnan E. Gout and the risk for incident heart failure and systolic dysfunction. *BMJ Open*. 2012;2:e000282.

35 Choi HK, Curhan G. Independent impact of gout on mortality and risk for coronary heart disease. *Circulation*. 2007;116:894-900.

36 Wright SA, Filippucci E, McVeigh C, et al. High resolution ultrasonography of the first metatarsal phalangeal joint in gout: a controlled study. *Ann Rheum Dis*. 2007;66:859-864.

37 Chen SY, Chen CL, Shen ML. Severity of gouty arthritis is associated with Q-wave myocardial infarction: a large-scale, cross-sectional study. *Clin Rheumatol*. 2007;26:308-313.

38 Perez-Ruiz F, Martinez-Indart L, Carmona L, Herrero-Beites AM, Pijoan JI, Krishnan E. Tophaceous gout and high level of hyperuricaemia are both associated with increased risk of mortality in patients with gout [published online ahead of print January 12, 2013]. Ann Rheum Dis. doi:10.1136/annrheumdis-2012-202421.

39 Pascual E, Castellano JA. Treatment with colchicine decreases white cell counts in synovial fluid of asymptomatic knees that contain monosodium urate crystals. *J Rheumatol*. 1992;19:600-603.

40 Crittenden DB, Lehmann RA, Schneck L, et al. Colchicine use is associated with decreased prevalence of myocardial infarction in patients with gout. *J Rheumatol*. 2012;39:1458-1464.

Chapter 3

Diagnosis of gout

Fernando Perez-Ruiz and Elena Garmendia

Introduction

A diagnosis of gout must be considered from different points of view, including epidemiologic, physiopathologic, and clinical. In addition, new imaging technologies have recently appeared as potential future diagnostic tools. Although several guidelines and recommendations have been published, neither the British Society for Rheumatology [1] nor the American College of Rheumatology (ACR) guidelines [2,3] have made any recommendations relating to gout diagnosis. So far, only the European League Against Rheumatism (EULAR) recommendations have taken diagnostic issues into consideration, and they state that monosodium urate crystal (MSUC) identification is the gold standard for diagnosis [4].

Classification criteria

Classification criteria were initially developed for epidemiologic use rather than for diagnosis. The American Rheumatology Association's (ARA, later ACR) "Preliminary Criteria for the Classification of the Acute Arthritis of Primary Gout" were developed for the classification of episodes of acute inflammation (EAIs) [5]. In addition, the authors clearly stated these preliminary criteria "to be useful in population surveys, and it seems appropriate to test them in the future in such an investigation," and that they should be further validated using a broad number of diseases (Table 3.1) [5]. On the contrary, these preliminary classification criteria

F. Perez-Ruiz and A. M. Herrero-Beites, *Managing Gout in Primary Care*, 25
DOI: 10.1007/978-1-907673-67-2_3, © Springer Healthcare 2014

Classification and diagnostic criteria

Criteria	Items		Limitations
ARA 1977 [5]: Major criteria or at least 6/12 minor criteria Sensitivity = 87% Specificity = 91%	Major	MSUCs in synovial fluid or a suspected tophus	Controls: RA, APPA, and septic arthritis
	Minor	1. Maximum inflammation develops within 1 day 2. More than one attack of acute arthritis 3. Monoarticular arthritis 4. Redness over joints 5. First MTP pain or swelling 6. Unilateral first MTP joint attack 7. Unilateral tarsal joint attack 8. Tophus (proven or suspected) 9. Hyperuricemia 10. Asymmetric swelling within a joint 11. Subcortical cysts, no erosions 12. Joint fluid culture negative for organisms	Not included: OA, spondyloarthropathies Other issues: Patients with septic arthritis and proven tophi Synovial fluid not available in most patients/controls Clinical data not available Retrospective data
Janssens et al 2010 [8]: Score <4 NPP 100% Score ≥8 PPV 80%	Item: 1. Male sex 2. Previous patient-reported arthritis attack 3. Onset within 1 day 4. Joint redness 5. MTP 1 involvement 6. Hypertension or ≥1 cardiovascular diseases 7. Serum uric acid level 5.88 mg/dL	Score: 2 2 0.5 1 2.5 1.5 3.5	Only patients with typical clinical presentation included: 100% only 1 joint involvement 57.4% first MTP involvement 85% ankle or foot involvement 89% erythema 89% men
	Maximum score	13	Not validated against other diseases

Table 3.1 Classification and diagnostic criteria. APPA=acute pyrophosphate arthritis; ARA=American Rheumatology Association; MSUCs=monosodium urate crystals; MTP=metatarsophalangeal; NPP=negative predictive value; OA=osteoarthritis; PPV=positive predictive value; RA=rheumatoid arthritis. Published with kind permission of © F. Perez-Ruiz 2014. All Rights Reserved.

for EAIs have often been inaccurately addressed as 'diagnostic' criteria for gout, independently of the clinical manifestations at the moment diagnosis was made. For example, a patient presenting with an EAI involving an ankle or knee joint for the first time does not qualify for clinical classification, and aspirating joints is strictly necessary for diagnosis.

These ARA criteria and the previous New York and Rome criteria were tested in a series of patients with gout using MSUCs in synovial fluid samples as a gold-standard comparator, with a sensitivity of 70%, 70%, and 67.7%, a specificity of 78.8%, 82.7%, and 88%, and a positive predictive value of 65.6%, 70%, and 76.9% reported, respectively [6]. Overall, the methodology used for the development of all these sets of classification criteria has been reported as poor [7].

Diagnostic criteria

The limited validity of the ARA criteria for the classification of gout was also demonstrated in the setting of MSUC-proven acute arthritis (sensitivity of 0.8 and specificity of 0.64) [8], and the authors of this study subsequently designed a diagnostic criteria set called "A Diagnostic Rule for Acute Gouty Arthritis in Primary Care Without Joint Fluid Analysis" [8]. The study was restricted to patients presenting with single-joint involvement, typical erythema (in most patients), and very frequent first metatarsophalangeal (MTP) involvement. In such typical clinical presentations, scorings of ≥8 using this diagnostic rule showed a specificity for gout diagnosis of 80%, whilst scorings <4 ruled out a diagnosis of gout in almost 100% of patients (Table 3.1) [9].

The question is whether physicians facing patients with typical clinical features of gout really need algorithms. Indeed, one study found that family physicians showed a concordance for diagnosis in 75% of patients' MSUC-proven gout and in 69% of patients showing >1 joint involvement, compared with 85% and 45%, respectively, for emergency room physicians and 30% and 42% for other specialists, with atypical presentation or long-term polyarticular involvement being the main source for discordance [10].

Typical acute, monoarticular joint involvement, mainly located in the first MTP or tarsal joints with accompanying erythema, show acceptable concordance with the gold-standard diagnosis [10]. Diagnosis accuracy is lower in 'atypical' presentations or long-term multiple joint involvement, and it should be taken into consideration that close to 20% of patients with gout will never suffer an EAI located in the first MTP joint.

Serum urate levels

Although hyperuricemia has been consistently included in classification and diagnostic criteria, serum urate (sUr) may be normal at the precise moment of the EAI in 10–40% of patients [11]. In addition, hyperuricemia is a frequent finding in adult populations, especially in the elderly. The EULAR recommendations advise that sUr levels may be normal in MSUC-proven gout, especially during acute inflammation in patients with normal renal function [4].

The presence or absence of hyperuricemia neither confirms nor rules out a diagnosis of gout. Therefore, sUr level has limited diagnostic value, especially for acute gout. To ascertain hyperuricemia, it is suggested that sUr levels be tested at least 1 or 2 weeks after an EAI.

Examination of synovial fluid

Since McCarty and Hollander found that MSUCs and calcium pyrophosphate dehydrate crystals (CPPCs) are present in the synovial fluid of patients with gout and pseudogout (acute pyrophosphate arthritis), and that MSUCs were different from CPPCs (by using a polarizing microscope) [12], there is a wide consensus that a definitive diagnosis of gout should be based on MSUC identification [4]. Unfortunately, obtaining synovial fluid samples requires training and skill to aspirate joints and the availability of a laboratory experienced in the detection and identification of crystals.

The EULAR recommendations suggest that aspiration of joints to obtain synovial fluid and examination under microscope during EAIs and also in the periods between EAIs (known as the 'intercritical period') should be considered for diagnosis [4]. In one study, after aspiration of knee joints, MSUCs were identified in 36/37 (97%) asymptomatic but previously inflamed knees [13]. Aspirating both symptomatic and asymptomatic first MTP joints yielded MSUCs in 73% and 58% of patients, respectively [14].

Monosodium urate crystals (MSUCs)

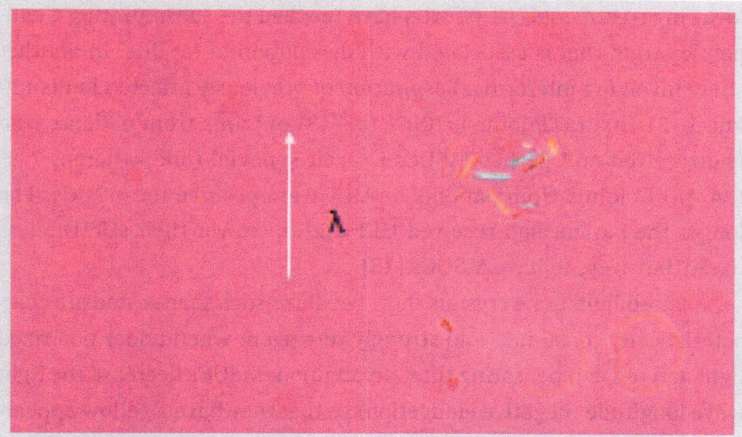

Figure 3.1 Monosodium urate crystals (MSUCs). Polarized light with red compensating filter, 400x. Small, non-acicular crystals are commonly observed in synovial fluid samples after the episode of acute inflammation has subsided. The MSUCs all show intense refringence, shine yellow when parallel to the polarizing axis (arrow, λ), and shine blue when perpendicular. Published with kind permission of © F. Perez-Ruiz 2014. All Rights Reserved.

Calcium pyrophosphate crystals (CPPCs)

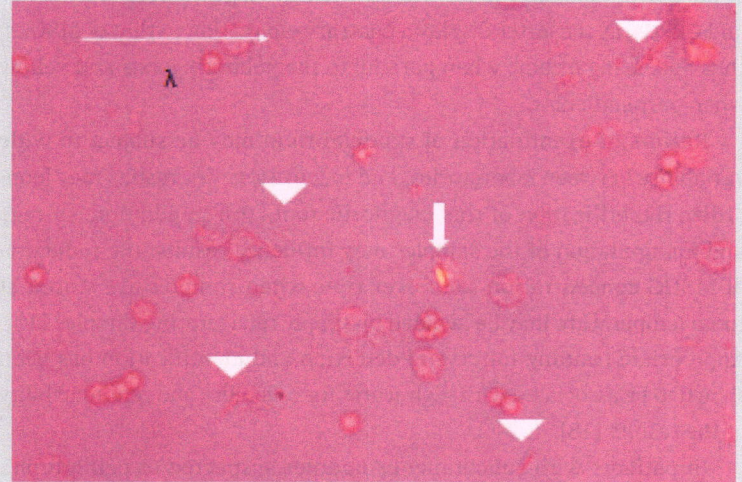

Figure 3.2 Calcium pyrophosphate crystals (CPPCs). Polarized light with red compensating filter, 400x. Most CPPCs are not refringent (arrow heads); some of them (arrow) show refringence and shine yellow when perpendicular to the polarizing axis, contrary to that displayed by MSUCs. Published with kind permission of © F. Perez-Ruiz 2014. All Rights Reserved.

These results may be lower in patients effectively treated with urate-lowering treatments (ULTs) who have reached the subsaturating therapeutic target that is associated with dissolution of MSUCs. In another study involving intercritical aspiration of previously affected joints (80 knees, 21 first MTP joints), 100% (43/43) of joints from patients who had received no ULT had MSUCs in their synovial fluid, whereas 71% (34/48) of joints from patients on ULT were positive for MSUCs. The longer the patient had received ULT and the lower their sUr, the less likely they were to have MSUCs [15].

Monosodium urate crystals show needle or stick shapes, and are characteristically constantly and strongly refringent when under polarized light and red compensating filter. In addition, MSUCs decrease the light wave longitude (negative elongation) so that they have a yellow appearance when parallel to the polarizing axis but blue when perpendicular to the polarizing axis (Figure 3.1). CPPCs may show either a paralepipedic (monoclinic crystallization) shape that may be confounded for MSUCs or a rhomboidal (triclinic crystallization) shape (Figure 3.2). Most of the monoclinic CPPCs are neither refringent nor weakly refringent; the use of polarizing light allows for the ability to distinguish between MSUCs and CPPCs, as the latter display a contrary elongation to that of MSUCs, thus appearing as blue when parallel to the polarizing axis and yellow when perpendicular.

Results of examination of synovial fluid may be subject to wide variability between laboratories, and inconsistency of results may jeopardize the utilization of this diagnostic tool [16]. In addition, storage and manipulation of the samples may influence results; the reduction of MSUC concentration seen over time when samples are stored at room temperature may be avoided by simply refrigerating samples [17]. Appropriate training for crystal detection and identification has been shown to be associated with high scores for reliability and reproducibility of the results [18].

In patients with subcutaneous nodules suspected of being tophi, puncture and aspiration may yield a whitish, chalk-like material that will show no cells but a myriad of MSUCs (Figure 3.3). Material obtained from draining tophi may also be used for microscopic examination.

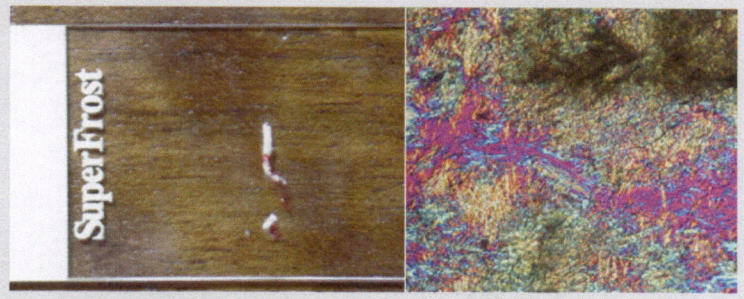

Macroscopic aspect of chalk-like material aspirated from a subcutaneous nodule suspected to be a tophus

Figure 3.3 Macroscopic aspect of chalk-like material aspirated from a subcutaneous nodule suspected to be a tophus. Polarized light with red compensating filter, 400x. Presence of thousands of MSUCs and absence of cells are evident. Published with kind permission of © F. Perez-Ruiz 2014. All Rights Reserved.

An issue of clinical importance is that septic arthritis and acute crystal-induced arthritis was found to occur simultaneously in up to 1–2% of patients who visited emergency rooms, as joints inflamed by crystals may become infected. Therefore, the presence of crystals cannot exclude septic arthritis with certainty [19]. Accurate clinical evaluation and sending samples to a laboratory for culture are mandatory when risk factors for infection, or symptoms or analysis suggestive of infection, are present.

Imaging techniques used in the assessment of gout

Gout was mostly evaluated with plain radiography until the recent appearance of new imaging techniques [20,21]. The use of ultrasonography, computed tomography (CT), magnetic resonance imaging (MRI), and most recently dual-energy CT (DECT) may help with diagnoses, particularly in evaluating and monitoring the burden of urate deposition [22].

Plain radiography

X-ray is not a sensitive or specific technique for the diagnosis of gout, as changes appear late in the natural history of disease; ultrasonography has been shown to be more sensitive than X-ray in early disease [21,23]. Therefore, systematic X-ray is not recommended for diagnosis or evaluation of patients initially presenting with gout.

X-ray subtle erosion in the lateral-dorsal aspect of the first metatarsal bone head with overhanging periosteal reaction, which was only appreciated in oblique projection

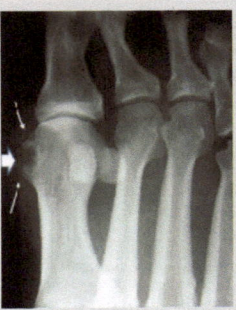

Figure 3.4 X-ray subtle erosion in the lateral-dorsal aspect of the first metatarsal bone head with overhanging periosteal reaction, which was only appreciated in oblique projection. Published with kind permission of © F. Perez-Ruiz 2014. All Rights Reserved.

X-ray extensive erosions and multiple joint destruction in a patient with widespread, 15-year-long gout

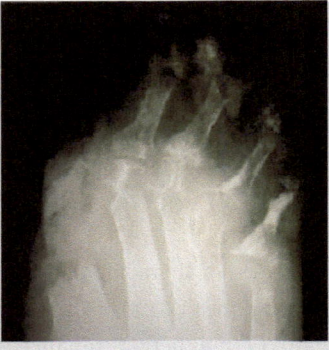

Figure 3.5 X-ray extensive erosions and multiple joint destruction in a patient with widespread, 15-year-long gout. The first toe had to be amputated due to severe tissue destruction and concomitant infection. Published with kind permission of © F. Perez-Ruiz 2014. All Rights Reserved.

Nevertheless, in patients with chronic or long-term intermittent joint disease, X-ray may help with differential diagnosis, especially to distinguish gout from calcium pyrophosphate arthritis if chondrocalcinosis is present and to confirm the need for synovial fluid analysis. Typical X-ray changes in late gout are considered to be highly specific and differentiate early versus late disease [24].

In early gout, only an increase in soft tissues may be evident during the EAIs. After repeated EAIs, well-defined bone erosions without surrounding osteopenia and with typical overhanging periosteal reaction may be evident; sometimes oblique projections may be needed to ascertain the presence of erosions (Figure 3.4). Patients with untreated or neglected gout will, through time, develop polyarticular, severe destructive joint disease (see Chapter 1) that is sometimes difficult to distinguish from other erosive chronic inflammatory diseases (Figure 3.5).

Patients treated to target subsaturating therapeutic sUr levels show a reduction in the number and size of bone erosions, but no change related to intra-articular structures [25], suggesting that presence of X-ray 'chronic gouty arthropathy' is a predictor of structural sequelae.

Ultrasonography

Ultrasonography has become a widely used imaging technique for diagnosis and evaluation of patients in clinical practice. A number of specialists and primary care practitioners commonly use ultrasonography in clinical practice due to its accuracy [26], feasibility, lower cost, and absence of radiation [22]. High-resolution ultrasonography is able to detect urate deposition in one in four patients with longstanding hyperuricemia even prior to the appearance of the very first symptom of gout [27,28].

Although findings such as synovial hypertrophy, power-doppler signal, or erosions are not specific for gout, some ultrasonography findings are highly specific [20]. The presence of the double contour sign (Figure 3.6) shows a specificity close to 100% and represents the deposition of urate

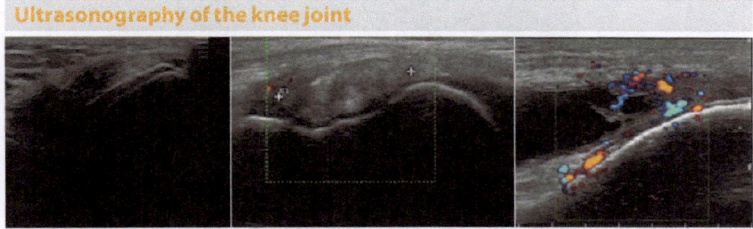

Ultrasonography of the knee joint

Figure 3.6 Ultrasonography of the knee joint. (a) Transverse, femoral condyle showing double contour sign; (b) Longitudinal, nodular hyperechoic nodule under the lateral ligament of the knee with peripheral power-doppler signal; (c) Longitudinal, suprapatellar bursae showing increased synovial thickness and intense power-doppler signalling. Published with kind permission of © F. Perez-Ruiz 2014. All Rights Reserved.

over the surface of the hyaline cartilage (see Figure 1.1 for an arthroscopic view), although the prevalence varies depending on the time
from onset of gout. Hyperechoic 'cloudy' areas within the synovium are
frequently found, with specificity being over 90% [23]. Bright dotted
foci and hyperechoic stippled aggregates are also very frequent, with
specificity being close to 75% [3]. From a clinical and practical point
of view, in patients with an uncertain diagnosis in whom gout could be
a plausible cause and with no availability for accurate synovial fluid
examination, an ultrasonographic examination showing highly specific
findings of MSUC deposition could be helpful.

High-resolution ultrasonography has been compared with MRI and is
validated to be accurate, reliable, and sensitive to change as an outcome
measure in patients treated with urate-lowering agents [29]. Although
not specific, the presence of inflammation in the joint structures or
peripheral to tophaceous aggregates can be assessed with power-doppler
imaging [22].

Computed tomography

Computed tomography findings in gout have been shown to be useful
for the detection of intra-osseous tophi (Figure 3.7), and correlate the
presence of erosions seen with X-ray [30]. However, in addition to being
nonspecific, expensive, and radioactive, its clinical use may be limited to

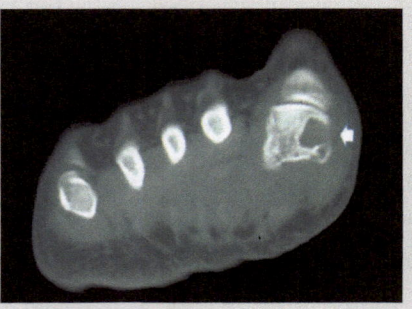

Figure 3.7 Computed tomography imaging showing an intraosseous tophus in the first
metatarsal head erosion (arrow) due to MSUC deposition. Published with kind permission of ©
F. Perez-Ruiz 2014. All Rights Reserved.

evaluating the possibility of gout involvement in atypical locations [31]. It has not been shown to perform better than physical measurement of tophi [32].

Dual-energy CT

Dual-energy CT is a sophisticated device that uses two beams as the source of radiation. It is able to differentiate MSUCs from calcium-containing crystals in tissues (as used for kidney stones); a large amount of interest has therefore recently arisen around this technique [33]. Currently, DECT is an expensive, not widely available, radiating procedure, to be considered mostly for investigation, clinical trials, or selected clinical cases.

Dual-energy CT has shown to be highly specific for MSUC deposition in bones, joints, and tendons [34], and some have even suggested that it could be the definitive imaging diagnostic tool [35]. A detailed analysis of recent evidence suggests that DECT findings are related to the burden of deposition, and DECT may be negative in patients with early gout [36].

Magnetic resonance imaging

Magnetic resonance imaging has shown nonspecific findings related to gout, though it is more sensitive to structural joint changes than X-ray [37]. It is useful for detecting tophi and MSUC deposition in joints and tendons, and also evaluates synovial thickness and inflammation using gadolinium enhancement (Figure 3.8). Magnetic resonance imaging

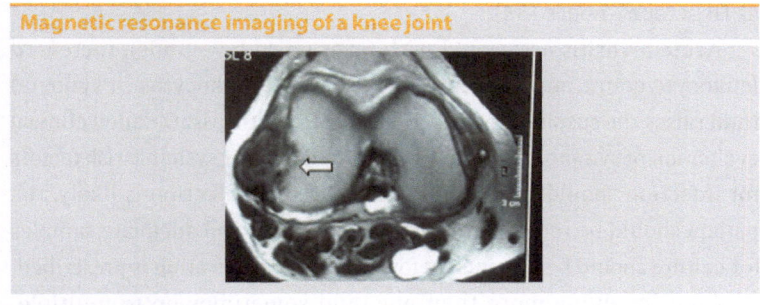

Magnetic resonance imaging of a knee joint

Figure 3.8 Magnetic resonance imaging of a knee joint. Magnetic resonance imaging of a knee joint showing extensive deposition of MSUCs in the lateral aspect (arrow) below the lateral ligament, with associated bone erosion of the femoral condyle. Extensive synovial thickening is also evident. Published with kind permission of © F. Perez-Ruiz 2014. All Rights Reserved.

may also be useful for differentiating symptoms caused by structural damage (meniscal tears, ligament derangements) from those caused by MSUC aggregates.

Chronic synovitis due to MSUC deposition is typically hypointense in T1- and T2-weighted sequences and may be confounded with granulomatous diseases (including tuberculosis), tumours (pigmented villonodular synovitis and synovial giant cell tumours), hemochromatosis, amyloid deposition, and siderosis due to intermittent bleeding [38].

Differential diagnosis

Typical gout, starting from the first MTP, with rapid onset, associated skin erythema over the involved joint, and showing adequate and rapid response to anti-inflammatory medication should not be a complicated clinical diagnosis. However, non-gouty bursitis, osteoarthritis, and stress fractures are commonly confused with gout in patients with hyperuricemia. Also, acute pyrophosphate arthritis involving the first MTP joint closely mimics gout, making diagnosis more difficult.

In the elderly, in whom the prevalence of hyperuricemia may be up to 20%, acute inflammation in the knee, ankle, wrist, or MTP joints may be due to acute pyrophosphate arthritis, and in some patients both MSUCs and CPPCs may be found in synovial fluid. In the elderly, gout more frequently appears in atypical locations, such as the fingers or wrists, and EAIs are more often polyarticular and may appear in previously osteoarthritic joints. Enlarging tophi are also commonly misdiagnosed as Heberden's nodes [39].

Acute arthritis associated with fever (even low-grade), increased leukocyte count in peripheral blood, or high leukocytes in synovial fluid raises the suspicion of infectious (septic) arthritis. Detailed clinical evaluation of symptoms, disease course, and local or systemic risk factors for infection should be carefully considered; if infection is likely, the patient should be referred for further evaluation and adequate samples for culture should be obtained before antibiotic medication is prescribed.

Gout involving more than one, and sometimes up to multiple, joints from onset may be confounded with spondyloarthropathies, the distribution of which are most frequently found asymmetrically in the lower limbs [40].

In the most severe cases, polyarticular symmetric involvement of hands and feet occasionally inducing swan-neck deformities, associated with subcutaneous nodules and showing extensive erosive disease in X-ray, may be confounded with rheumatoid arthritis (Figure 3.9) [41].

Polyarticular joint involvement of the hands, with swan-neck deformities and sustained chronic inflammation

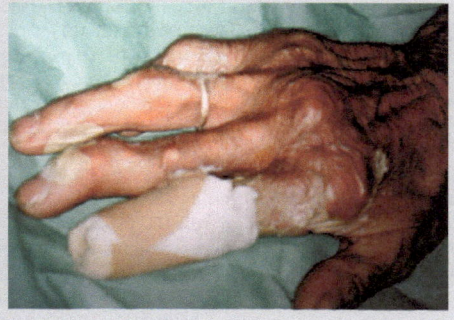

Figure 3.9 Polyarticular joint involvement of the hands, with swan-neck deformities and sustained chronic inflammation. The patient had been previously treated with methotrexate and azathioprine for rheumatoid arthritis (see evolution pictures in Chapter 4). Published with kind permission of © F. Perez-Ruiz 2014. All Rights Reserved.

Key points

- Classification criteria should not be considered to be diagnostic criteria.
- Diagnostic criteria developed for general practitioners lack extrinsic applicability to atypical presentations.
- Appropriate diagnosis is based on MSUC observation by microscopy.
- Imaging techniques, particularly ultrasound, may show highly specific findings and be of special interest in evaluating the burden of deposition and its response to treatment in selected patients.
- Differential diagnosis should be always kept in mind in patients with hyperuricemia and arthritis.

References

1   Jordan KM, Cameron JS, Snaith M, et al; on behalf of the British Society for Rheumatology and British Health Professionals in Rheumatology Standards, Guidelines and Audit Working Group (SGAWG). British Society for Rheumatology and British Health Professionals in Rheumatology guideline for the management of gout. *Rheumatology (Oxford)*. 2007;46:1372-1374.

2   Khanna D, Fitzgerald JD, Khanna PP, et al. 2012 American College of Rheumatology guidelines for management of gout. Part 1: Systematic nonpharmacologic and pharmacologic therapeutic approaches to hyperuricemia. *Arthritis Care Res (Hoboken)*. 2012;64:1431-1446.

3   Khanna D, Khanna PP, Fitzgerald JD, et al. 2012 American College of Rheumatology guidelines for management of gout. Part 2: Therapy and antiinflammatory prophylaxis of acute gouty arthritis. *Arthritis Care Res (Hoboken)*. 2012;64:1447-1461.

4   Zhang W, Doherty M, Pascual E, et al. EULAR evidence based recommendations for gout. Part I. Diagnosis. Report of a task force of the Standing Committee for International Clinical Studies Including Therapeutics (ESCISIT). *Ann Rheum Dis*. 2006;65:1301-1311.

5   Wallace SL, Robinson H, Masi AT, Decker JL, McCarty DJ, Yü TF. Preliminary criteria for the classification of the acute arthritis of primary gout. *Arthritis Rheum*. 1977;20:895-900.

6   Malik A, Schumacher HR, Dinnella JE, Clayburne GM. Clinical diagnostic criteria for gout: comparison with the gold standard of synovial fluid crystal analysis. *J Clin Rheumatol*. 2009;15:22-24.

7   Johnson SR, Goek O-N, Singh-Grewal D, et al. Classification criteria in rheumatic diseases: a review of methodologic properties. *Arthritis Rheum*. 2007;57:1119-1133.

8   Janssens HJEM, Fransen J, van de Lisdonk EH, van Riel PLCM, van Weel C, Janssen M. A diagnostic rule for acute gouty arthritis in primary care without joint fluid analysis. *Arch Intern Med*. 2010;170:1120-1126.

9   Janssens HJEM, Janssen M, van de Lisdonk EH, Fransen J, van Riel PLCM, van Weel C. Limited validity of the American College of Rheumatology criteria for classifying patients with gout in primary care. *Ann Rheum Dis*. 2010;69:1255-1256.

10 Pérez Ruiz F, Ruiz López J, Herrero Beites AM. Influence of the natural history of disease on a previous diagnosis in patients with gout . *Reumatol Clin*. 2009;5:248-251.

11 Leiszler M, Poddar S, Fletcher A. Clinical inquiry. Are serum uric acid levels always elevated in acute gout? *J Fam Pract*. 2011;60:618-620.

12 McCarty DJ, Hollander JL. Identification of urate crystals in gouty synovial fluid. *Ann Intern Med*. 1961;54:452-460.

13 Pascual E. Persistence of monosodium urate crystals and low-grade inflammation in synovial fluid of patients with untreated gout. *Arthritis Rheum*. 1991;34:141-145.

14 Sivera F, Aragon R, Pascual E. First metatarsophalangeal joint aspiration using a 29-gauge needle. *Ann Rheum Dis*. 2008;67:273-275.

15 Pascual E, Batlle-Gualda E, Martínez A, Rosas J, Vela P. Synovial fluid analysis for diagnosis of intercritical gout. *Ann Intern Med*. 1999;131:756-759.

16 Amer H, Swan A, Dieppe P. The utilization of synovial fluid analysis in the UK. *Rheumatology (Oxford)*. 2001;40:1060-1063.

17 Graf SW, Buchbinder R, Zochling J, Whittle SL. The accuracy of methods for urate crystal detection in synovial fluid and the effect of sample handling: a systematic review. *Clin Rheumatol*. 2013;32:225-232.

18 Lumbreras B, Pascual E, Frasquet J, González-Salinas J, Rodriguez E, Hernández-Aguado I. Analysis for crystals in synovial fluid: training of the analysts results in high consistency. *Ann Rheum Dis*. 2005;64:612-615.

19 Shah K, Spear J, Nathanson LA, McCauley J, Edlow JA. Does the presence of crystal arthritis rule out septic arthritis? *J Emerg Med*. 2007;32:23-26.

20 Perez-Ruiz F, Dalbeth N, Urresola A, de Miguel E, Schlesinger N. Imaging of gout: findings and utility. *Arthritis Res Ther*. 2009;11:232.

21 Wright SA, Filippucci E, McVeigh C, et al. High resolution ultrasonography of the first metatarsal phalangeal joint in gout: a controlled study. *Ann Rheum Dis.* 2007;66:859-864.

22 Perez-Ruiz F, Naredo E. Imaging modalities and monitoring measures of gout. *Curr Opin Rheumatol.* 2007;19:128-133.

23 Rettenbacher T, Ennemoser S, Weirich H, et al. Diagnostic imaging of gout: comparison of high-resolution US versus conventional X-ray. Eur J Radiol. 2008;18:621-630.

24 Dalbeth N, Clark B, McQueen F, Doyle A, Taylor W. Validation of a radiographic damage index in chronic gout. *Arthritis Rheum.* 2007;57:1067-1073.

25 Bloch C, Hermann G, Yu T-F. A radiologic reevaluation of gout: a study of 2,000 patients. AJR *Am J Roentgenol.* 1980;134:781-787.

26 Howard RG, Pillinger MH, Gyftopoulos S, Thiele RG, Swearingen CJ, Samuels J. Reproducibility of musculoskeletal ultrasound for determining monosodium urate deposition: concordance between readers. *Arthritis Care Res (Hoboken).* 2011;63:1456-1462.

27 De Miguel E, Puig JG, Castillo C, Peiteado D, Torres RJ, Martín-Mola E. Diagnosis of gout in patients with asymptomatic hyperuricemia: a pilot ultrasound study. *Ann Rheum Dis.* 2012;71:157-158.

28 Pineda C, Amezcua-Guerra LM, Solano C, et al. Joint and tendon subclinical involvement suggestive of gouty arthritis in asymptomatic hyperuricemia: an ultrasound controlled study. *Arthritis Res Ther.* 2011;13:R4.

29 Perez-Ruiz F, Martin I, Canteli B. Ultrasonographic measurement of tophi as an outcome measure for chronic gout. *J Rheumatol.* 2007;34:1888-1893.

30 Dalbeth N, Clark B, Gregory K, et al. Mechanisms of bone erosions in gout: a quantitative analysis using plain radiography and computed tomography. *Ann Rheum Dis.* 2009;68:1290-1295.

31 Konatalapalli RM, Lumezanu E, Jelinek JS, Murphey MD, Wang H, Weinstein A. Correlates of axial gout: a cross-sectional study. *J Rheumatol.* 2012;39:1445-1449.

32 Dalbeth N, Clark B, Gregory K, Gamble GD, Doyle A, McQueen FM. Computed tomography measurement of tophus volume: comparison with physical measurement. *Arthritis Rheum.* 2007;57:461-465.

33 Artmann A, Ratzenböck M, Noszian I, Trieb K. Dual energy CT–a new perspective in the diagnosis of gout. *Rofo.* 2010;182:261-266.

34 Glazebrook KN, Guimarães LS, Murthy NS, et al. Identification of intraarticular and periarticular uric acid crystals with dual-energy CT: initial evaluation. *Radiology.* 2011;261:516-524.

35 Nicolaou S, Yong-Hing CJ, Galea-Soler S, Hou DJ, Louis L, Munk P. Dual-energy CT as a potential new diagnostic tool in the management of gout in the acute setting. *AJR Am J Roentgenol.* 2010;194:1072-1078.

36 McQueen FM, Doyle AJ, Reeves Q, Gamble GD, Dalbeth N. DECT urate deposits: now you see them, now you don>t. *Ann Rheum Dis.* 2012;72:458-459.

37 Carter JD, Kedar RP, Anderson SR, et al. An analysis of MRI and ultrasound imaging in patients with gout who have normal plain radiographs. *Rheumatology (Oxford).* 2009;48:1442-1446.

38 Narváez JA, Narváez J, Ortega R, De Lama E, Roca Y, Vidal N. Hypointense synovial lesions on T2-weighted images: differential diagnosis with pathologic correlation. *AJR Am J Roentgenol.* 2003;181:761-769.

39 Campbell SM. Gout: how presentation, diagnosis, and treatment differ in the elderly. *Geriatrics.* 1988;43:71-77.

40 Wolfe F, Cathey MA. The misdiagnosis of gout and hyperuricemia. *J Rheumatol.* 1991;18:1232-1234.

41 Perez-Ruiz F, Ruiz Lopez J, Herrero Beites A. Influence of the natural history of disease on a previous diagnosis in patients with gout. *Rheumatol Clin.* 2009;5:248-251.

Chapter 4

Treatment of hyperuricemia in gout

Fernando Perez-Ruiz and Joana Atxotegi

Introduction

The treatment of gout with chronic clinical manifestations comprises three aspects, in the following order of clinical importance: 1) reducing serum urate to the therapeutic range to dissolve monosodium urate crystals (MSUCs) formed in tissues, using urate-lowering therapy (ULT); 2) preventing or reducing the risk of episodes of acute inflammation (EAIs) that appear and even increase in frequency during the initiation of ULT (prophylaxis); 3) promptly, safely, and effectively treating any EAIs that may appear until proper and stable serum urate levels are achieved. As they are intimately linked, the last two points will be discussed in the next chapter.

Indications for urate-lowering therapy

ULT comprises any measure implemented to reduce serum urate levels (sUr) to a subsaturating, therapeutic target. Thus, ULT is indicated in all patients with a definite diagnosis of gout. A nonpharmacologic approach to correct hyperuricemia, implementing lifestyle changes if applicable, should be considered for any patient. Urate-lowering medications (ULMs) should then be considered in patients in whom nonpharmacologic measures are either not applicable or not effective [1].

The European League Against Rheumatism (EULAR) 2006 recommendations suggest that pharmacologic ULT should be started in patients

F. Perez-Ruiz and A. M. Herrero-Beites, *Managing Gout in Primary Care*, 41
DOI: 10.1007/978-1-907673-67-2_4, © Springer Healthcare 2014

showing recurrent episodes of inflammation, tophi, arthropathy or X-ray lesions [2], while the 2012 guidelines from the American College of Rheumatology (ACR) recommend ULT for patients in whom tophi are present or who have more than two EAIs per year [3]. The ACR guidelines also suggest ULT in those who have previous urolithiasis or who have chronic kidney disease stage 2 or worse [3].

In some infrequent instances, patients may have sUr in the therapeutic range and crystal-proven gout, as is the case of patients with previous but not actual hyperuricemia due to previous diuretic treatment or after considerable weight loss or reduction of heavy alcohol use. For such patients, a period of prophylaxis and treatment for the EAIs should be prescribed [4].

Targets for urate-lowering therapy

Different therapeutic sUr targets should be considered depending on the extent of MSUC deposition, mainly based on the presence of subcutaneous or articular tophi or polyarticular distribution of joint involvement. Consistently lowering sUr to the therapeutic target is associated with a progressive reduction and disappearance of subcutaneous and articular tophi and a decreased rate of flares, to almost zero over the long term [5]. Indeed, sUr during ULT may be considered as a biomarker for successful therapy [6].

In general, the therapeutic sUr target is <6 mg/dL (<360 μmol/L), which is lower than the saturation threshold for urate at close to 7 mg/dL or 420 μmol/L. This is in order to promote spontaneous dissolution of MSUCs. [2,3]

For patients with severe gout, it has been shown that there is an inverse relationship between sUr levels during therapy and the velocity of reduction of subcutaneous and articular tophi [7,8]. In other words, the lower the sUr, the better for reducing deposition of severe gout (Figure 4.1). This differentiation of sUr targets, depending on the burden of disease, has been included in the ACR guidelines for the treatment of gout [3].

Once MSUC deposits are completely dissolved, there is no real need to keep sUr as low as the therapeutic targets. They can be kept just below the saturation threshold in order to avoid new MSUC formation, which is the sUr target for secondary prevention [9].

Extensive tophaceous deposition in the joints of the hands, and disappearance of tophi after ULT with average serum urate levels <4 mg/dL (<240 µmol/L)

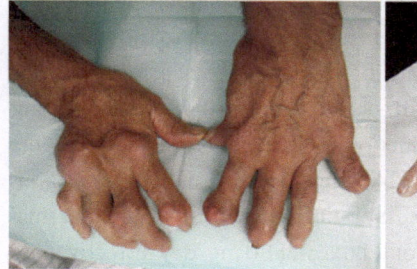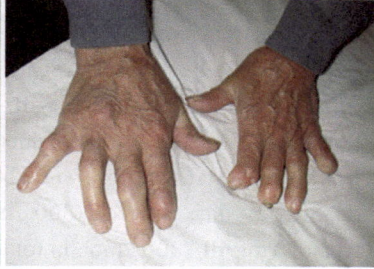

Figure 4.1 Extensive tophaceous deposition in the joints of the hands, and disappearance of tophi after ULT with average serum urate levels <4 mg/dL (<240 µmol/L). Published with kind permission of © F. Perez-Ruiz 2014. All Rights Reserved.

Nonpharmacological approach to the treatment of hyperuricemia: lifestyle modification

There is limited evidence regarding the impact of lifestyle change on the reduction of sUr in patients with gout, but such changes have been shown to be of some benefit with regard to the reduction of factors associated with risk of cardiovascular events.

The correction of overweight or obesity is certainly beneficial for general health, but weight loss >10 kg did not produce the anticipated reduction in sUr, with a reduction of just over 1 mg/dL (60 μmol/L) on average [10]. The 2010 US Department of Agriculture and Department of Health and Human Services dietary guidelines outline healthy eating patterns that are also applicable to patients with gout [11]. An advisable diet would be one with more vegetable or dairy protein than animal protein, cereals as a main source of complex sugars, and restriction of salt, alcoholic beverages, and sweetmeals [11].

In patients concomitantly treated with medications known to induce or contribute to hyperuricemia, such as thiazides in patients with hypertension, the use of alternative antihypertensive drugs, in particular losartan due to the mild uricosuric effect that it exerts, should be considered [2]. Withdrawal of diuretics would not be an option to consider for patients taking these agents due to them suffering from chronic kidney disease or chronic heart failure [2].

Pharmacological management

Selection of urate-lowering drugs

There are some factors that should be considered when prescribing ULMs. Availability of these agents may differ from one country to the other, and labels may also be different regarding indications or dosing. Efficacy, defined as the reduction in mg/dL per dose prescribed, varies among ULMs. The estimated a priori reduction of sUr from baseline in patients with normal renal function would be 3 mg/dL (180 μmol/L) for allopurinol 300 mg/day, 5 mg/dL (300 μmol/L) for benzbromarone 100 mg/day, and 5 mg/dL (300 μmol/L) for febuxostat 80 mg/day. Effectiveness is considered to be the percentage of patients reaching therapeutic sUr target at a given dose, and is dependent on baseline sUr and ULM efficacy [12]. For patients averaging baseline sUr 9 mg/dL (540 μmol/L), 85% to 90% effectiveness will be reached with allopurinol 600 mg/day, benzbromarone 100 mg/day, or febuxostat 80 mg/day [13]. Safety should also be considered, as should the clinical profile of the patient, including comorbidities (especially kidney and liver function). Concomitant medications that may show pharmacokinetic interactions with ULMs should be carefully analyzed prior to starting ULMs.

Clinical experience, guidelines, and proper communication with the patient can all help physicians to individually schedule ULT and, if needed, to refer to or consult with a colleague or specialist with advanced experience in treating difficult-to-treat gout.

Urate-lowering medications

The term ULM includes any drug that shows an effect on lowering sUr. They may act through one of three different mechanisms: inhibition of xanthine-oxidoreductase (XOR), reducing endogenous uric acid production (allopurinol and febuxostat); inhibition of renal tubular transporters that reabsorb uric acid, thus enhancing uric acid excretion or 'uricosuria' (benzbromarone, sulphinpyrazone, and probenecid); or breakdown of uric acid to alantoin (pegloticase and other uricases) [12].

Initiation of ULM

It is advised to "start (at) low (doses) and go slow" with progressive increases of ULM doses [2]. Doses should not be increased within a 2-week period. It is also recommended not to change the dose (increase, decrease, or withdraw) of ULM during an EAI flare or escalate doses if the sUr target is still to be achieved until the flare has completely subsided. Patients should be aware of the risk of flaring during the first year of ULM and avoid withdrawing from ULM.

The ULM dose should be raised until the therapeutic sUr target is reached (within approved doses) or to the maximum medically adequate dose for safety. It has been shown that over 50% of patients with gout with normal kidney function will reach the therapeutic sUr target with allopurinol 300 mg/day, febuxostat 80 mg/day, probenecid 1500 mg/day, or benzbromarone 50 mg/day; it is appropriate to check sUr at such doses and escalate the dose if further sUr reduction is needed [4].

In addition, starting treatment to prevent the development of EAIs should be carefully considered when initiating ULT, and especially ULMs. Also, patients should be prescribed ULMs in a way that potential EAIs can be readily treated.

Allopurinol

Allopurinol is a pro-drug that is metabolized and converted into active metabolites, oxypurinol being the main one. Oxypurinol exerts an inhibiting effect on the reduced isoform of XOR and is mostly excreted through the kidney, so its kinetics are modified with loss of renal function. The maximum approved dose of allopurinol varies widely, but in some countries it may be up to 900 mg/day for severe cases. However, in surveys [14] and an audit [15] of patients with gout it was uncommon to find patients who were on doses >300 mg/day.

The efficacy of allopurinol in reducing sUr levels has been estimated to be close to a reduction of 1 mg/dL (60 μmol/L) for every 100 mg/day in patients with normal renal function [12,15]. Increasing the dose of allopurinol from 300 mg/day is associated with a further decrease of sUr. Data from the only published double-blind, randomized, parallel, actively controlled clinical trial with high doses of allopurinol show that the average reduction of sUr for allopurinol was 3.3 mg/dL (198 μmol/L) (33% from a baseline of 9 mg/dL) with 300 mg/day and 4.5 mg/dL (270 μmol/L) (49% from baseline) in patients whose dose was increased to 600 mg/day for two months [14,16].

It is advised that the maximum doses of allopurinol to be reached should be adjusted and reduced (depending on renal function) to avoid an increase in the risk of severe adverse events [2]. Standard correction of allopurinol doses were based on empiric recommendations [17], and it has been shown that such dose correction led to improper sUr control in most patients [18]. Starting from a low dose and going up to 6 mg/day per unit of glomerular filtration rate (GFR; mg/mL/min) has been reported to not be associated with increased risk of serious adverse events [19].

A higher starting dose of allopurinol has also been associated with an increase in adverse events in patients with chronic renal disease. Recently it has been suggested that a starting dose of <1.5 mg/day per unit of GFR is associated with a reduced risk of adverse events [20].

Taking into consideration all the factors relating to renal function, overall allopurinol is a safe drug. The most common adverse reactions observed are altered liver function tests and mild skin rash [21]. Nevertheless, previous skin reactions, diuretic use, reduced GFR, initially uncorrected doses, and genetic predisposition are risk factors for developing serious adverse events, including Stevens-Johnson syndrome [22] and Drug-Related Eosinophilia with Systemic Symptoms (DRESS) [23], which includes what was previously known as 'allopurinol hypersensitivity syndrome.' A study by Lonjou et al. demonstrated the presence of the HLA-B*5801 allele in half the cases of allopurinol-induced severe cutaneous adverse reactions, in Caucasian patients [24].

Febuxostat

Febuxostat is approved in a number of countries, including the European Union, the United States, and Japan, for the treatment of hyperuricemia in patients with gout, although approved doses vary. It is a selective inhibitor of both isoforms of XOR, and is associated with an intense, linear, and dose-dependent reduction of sUr at standard doses [25].

Febuxostat is highly bioavailable after oral dosing. It has been shown to not significantly interact with drugs frequently used by patients with gout, such as thiazides, nonsteroidal anti-inflammatory drugs, and anticoagulants, and no dose correction is needed in patients with mild-to-moderate reduction of the GFR or mild liver dysfunction, namely Child-Pugh A stage level of liver disease [26]. To date, there are no clinical trial data for febuxostat treatment in patients with severe chronic kidney disease, dialysis, or solid organ transplants, which suggests that febuxostat should not be recommended in these patients.

In clinical trials, febuxostat 80 mg/day demonstrated an average sUr reduction of 4.5 mg/dL (270 μmol/L) (46% from a baseline of 9.8 mg/dL [588 μmol/L]) [12]. Furthermore, the effectiveness (the percentage of patients whose sUr was lower than the therapeutic target of 6 mg/dL at the final visit) of febuxostat 80 mg/day was superior to allopurinol 300 mg/day in two Phase 3 clinical trials (74% vs. 36% [27], and 67% vs. 42% [28], respectively).

An open-label extension study involving patients from one of the above Phase 3 clinical trials allowed patients who failed to reach therapeutic target in one arm of the study to change to the other arm of therapy. Over half of the patients initially assigned to take allopurinol were changed to febuxostat, while only one in five assigned to febuxostat 80 mg/day had to be reassigned to the other arm of treatment [29]. Sustained and long-term control of sUr levels to therapeutic target was associated with a progressive decline in the number of EAIs and a reduction in the rate of the presence of subcutaneous tophi [29,30].

In patients failing to reach therapeutic target, increasing the dose from 80 to 120 mg/day (a dose not currently approved in the US) may allow better control of sUr levels [27,29].

Uricosuric agents

Uricosuric agents are infrequently prescribed; sulfinpyrazone is unavailable or has been withdrawn from the market in most countries and benzbromarone is not available worldwide (and never has been in the US), and in addition has been restricted in most countries of the European Union. Probenecid is still available in some countries.

All of the above-mentioned agents increase renal excretion of uric acid into the urine by inhibiting tubular transporters that enhance reabsorption of uric acid. Whereas benzbromarone has been shown to be a potent inhibitor of URAT1 renal tubular transporter, with remarkable efficacy in reducing sUr [29,31] even in patients who have moderate renal function impairment [32], who are on diuretics, and who are on renal transplant medications [33], sulfinpyrazone and probenecid are less potent uricosurics and exert only a mild-to-moderate reduction of sUr, an effect that is supposed to be blunted in patients with moderate renal function impairment, contrary to the data reported in a recent retrospective study [34].

Pegloticase for severe chronic refractory gout

Failure to adequately control sUr levels ('treatment-failure gout') is observed in clinical practice surveys and research. In most cases it is due to inadequate compliance, underdosage of ULMs, not reaching therapeutic target, or failure to consider target sUr to be under the 'normal' level [35]. Refractory gout is defined as the clinical situation in which a persistence of gout symptoms is associated with improper control of sUr once all the available ULMs have been implemented to the maximal doses labelled or tolerated, or when adverse events limit or contraindicate the prescription of effective doses of ULMs [36].

Pegloticase (polyethylene-glycol-uricase) is a recombinant uricase conjugated to poly(ethylene glycol) to augment its half-life and reduce immunogenicity [37]. It was first approved by the US Food and Drug Administration and recently by the European Medicines Agency (EMA) for the treatment of severe refractory chronic gout ." The EMA label recommends that treatment with pegloticase be initiated and supervised by physicians who specialize in the diagnosis and treatment of severe refractory chronic gout [38].

Pegloticase is administered intravenously at a dose of 8 mg every other week. Infusion reactions are not infrequent, and have been associated with the development of circulating antibodies to the drug and clinically associated with lack of response or loss of efficacy, which happens in most cases during the first 3 months of therapy [39]. To date, pegloticase should not be administered with other concomitant ULMs, and should be withdrawn when consecutive pre-infusion sUr levels are shown to be twice >6 mg/dL (360 μmol/L) [38].

Antibodies to pegloticase may appear early during the treatment and in up to 89% of patients [39]. Less than 2% of patients with a high titer of antibodies against pegloticase maintained urate-lowering effectiveness; such cases were associated with the highest incidence of infusion reactions. A posthoc analysis showed that loss of effectiveness preceded the first infusion reaction in over 90% of patients on the approved dose [39]. Therefore, EMA recommendations are to withdraw therapy with pegloticase in patients showing no response or loss of effectiveness, defined as pre-infusion serum urate levels >6 mg/dL initially or twice consecutively during follow-up, respectively.

Other treatments

Fenofibrate, losartan, and atorvastatin have been found to induce a mild uricosuric effect and reduce sUr levels 10–15% from baseline [40]. Therefore, these ULMs may be useful as adjuvant concomitant medications in patients with hypertriglyceridemia, hypertension, and hypercholesterolemia, respectively.

Surgery for gout may be considered to treat complications, such as infected subcutaneous tophi, nerve compressions, or joint replacement. In no case would surgical removal of tophi preclude the need for a comprehensive, individualized, and complete approach to the treatment of hyperuricemia.

Key points

- The ultimate aim of gout treatment is to completely dissolve deposits of MSUCs that are responsible of the clinical manifestations of gout.
- Correction of sUr well below the saturation threshold will lead to the dissolution of MSUCs.
- The target sUr for the treatment of hyperuricemia of gout is <6 mg/dL (<360 μmol/L); further reduction below 5 mg/dL (300 μmol/L) may be initially considered for patients with the most severe disease.
- ULT comprises both lifestyle and pharmacologic measures to reduce sUr to target.
- Several drugs or drug combinations may be considered to get to target sUr; the selection will depend on the patient's clinical experience and local labelling and recommendations.

References

1. Perez-Ruiz F. Treating to target: an strategy to cure gout. *Rheumatology (Oxford)*. 2009;48(suppl 2):ii9-ii14.
2. Zhang W, Doherty M, Bardin T, et al. EULAR evidence based recommendations for gout. Part II. Management. Report of a task force of the EULAR Standing Committee for International Clinical Studies Including Therapeutics (ESCISIT). *Ann Rheum Dis*. 2006;65:1312-1324.
3. Khanna D, Fitzgerald JD, Khanna PP, et al. 2012 American College of Rheumatology guidelines for management of gout. Part 1: Systematic nonpharmacologic and pharmacologic therapeutic approaches to hyperuricemia. *Arthritis Care Res (Hoboken)*. 2012;64:1431-1446.
4. Perez-Ruiz F, Schlesinger N. Management of gout. *Scand J Rheumatol*. 2008;37:81- 89.
5. Perez-Ruiz F, Lioté F. Lowering serum uric acid levels: what is the optimal target for improving clinical outcomes in gout? *Arthritis Rheum*. 2007;57:1324-1328.
6. Stamp LK, Zhu X, Dalbeth N, Jordan S, Edwards NL, Taylor W. Serum urate as a soluble biomarker in chronic gout—evidence that serum urate fulfills the OMERACT validation criteria for soluble biomarkers. *Semin Arthritis Rheum*. 2011;40:483-500.
7. Perez-Ruiz F, Calabozo M, Pijoan JI, Herrero-Beites AM, Ruibal A. Effect of urate-lowering therapy on the velocity of size reduction of tophi in chronic gout. *Arthritis Rheum*. 2002;47:356-360.
8. Perez-Ruiz F, Martin I, Canteli B. Ultrasonographic measurement of tophi as an outcome measure for chronic gout. *J Rheumatol*. 2007;34:1888-1893.
9. Perez-Ruiz F, Herrero-Beites AM, Carmona L. A two-stage approach to the treatment of hyperuricemia in gout: the "dirty dish" hypothesis. *Arthritis Rheum*. 2011;63:4002-4006.
10. Choi HK. Dietary risk factors for rheumatic diseases. *Curr Opin Rheumatol*. 2005;17:141-146.
11. U.S. Department of Agriculture and U.S. Department of Health and Human Services. Dietary Guidelines for Americans, 2010. 7th Edition. Washington, DC: U.S. Government Printing Office; 2010. http://www.health.gov/dietaryguidelines/dga2010/dietaryguidelines2010.pdf. Accessed May 16, 2013.

12. Perez Ruiz F, Herrero-Beites AM. Evaluation and treatment of gout as a chronic disease. Adv Ther. 2012;29:935-946.
13. Jansen TL, Richette P, Perez-Ruiz F, et al. International position paper on febuxostat. Clin Rheumatol. 2010;29:835-840.
14. Annemans L, Spaepen E, Gaskin M, et al. Gout in the UK and Germany: prevalence, comorbidities and management in general practice 2000-2005. Ann Rheum Dis. 2008;67: 960-966.
15. Perez-Ruiz F, Carmona L, Yebeñes MJG, et al; on behalf of the GEMA Study Group, Sociedad Española de Reumatología. An audit of the variability of diagnosis and management of gout in the rheumatology setting: the Gout Evaluation and Management study. J Clin Rheumatol. 2011;17:349-355.
16. Reinders MK, Haagsma C, Jansen TLThA, et al. A randomised controlled trial on the efficacy and tolerability with dose escalation of allopurinol 300–600 mg/day versus benzbromarone 100–200 mg/day in patients with gout. Ann Rheum Dis. 2009;68:892-897.
17. Hande KR, Noone RM, Stone WJ. Severe allopurinol toxicity: description and guidelines for prevention in patients with renal insufficiency. Am J Med. 1984;76:47-56.
18. Dalbeth N, Kumar S, Stamp L, Gow P. Dose adjustment of allopurinol according to creatinine clearance does not provide adequate control of hyperuricemia in patients with gout. J Rheumatol. 2006;33:1646-1650.
19. Perez-Ruiz F, Hernando I, Villar I, Nolla JM. Correction of allopurinol dosing should be based on clearance of creatinine, but not plasma creatinine levels: another insight to allopurinol-related toxicity. J Clin Rheumatol. 2005;11:129-133.
20. Stamp LK, Taylor WJ, Jones PB, et al. Starting dose is a risk factor for allopurinol hypersensitivity syndrome: a proposed safe starting dose of allopurinol. Arthritis Rheum. 2012;64:2529-2536.
21. Rundles RW, Metz EN, Silberman HR. Allopurinol in the treatment of gout. Ann Intern Med. 1966;64:229-268.
22. Mockenhaupt M, Viboud C, Dunant A, et al. Stevens-Johnson syndrome and toxic epidermal necrolysis: assessment of medication risks with emphasis on recently marketed drugs. The EuroSCAR-study. J Invest Dermatol. 2008;128:35-44.
23. Cacoub P, Musette P, Descamps V, et al. The DRESS syndrome: a literature review. Am J Med. 2011;124:588-597.
24. Lonjou C, Borot N, Sekula P, et al. A European study of HLA-B in Stevens-Johnson syndrome and toxic epidermal necrolysis related to five high-risk drugs. Pharmacogenet Genomics. 2008;18:99-107.
25. Khosravan R, Grabowski BA, Wu JT, Joseph-Ridge N, Vernillet L. Pharmacokinetics, pharmacodynamics and safety of febuxostat, a non-purine selective inhibitor of xanthine oxidase, in a dose escalation study in healthy subjects. Clin Pharmacokinet. 2006;45:821-841.
26. Perez-Ruiz F, Dalbeth N, Schlesinger N. Febuxostat, a novel drug for the treatment of hyperuricemia of gout. Future Rheumatol. 2008;3:421-427.
27. Becker MA, Schumacher HR Jr, Wortmann RL, et al. Febuxostat compared with allopurinol in patients with hyperuricemia and gout. N Engl J Med. 2005;353:2450-2461.
28. Becker MA, Schumacher HR, Espinoza LR, et al. The urate-lowering efficacy and safety of febuxostat in the treatment of the hyperuricemia of gout: the CONFIRMS trial. Arthritis Res Ther. 2010;12:R63.
29. Becker MA, Schumacher HR, MacDonald PA, Lloyd E, Lademacher C. Clinical efficacy and safety of successful longterm urate lowering with febuxostat or allopurinol in subjects with gout. J Rheumatol. 2009;36:1282.
30. Schumacher HR Jr, Becker MA, Lloyd E, MacDonald PA, Lademacher C. Febuxostat in the treatment of gout: 5-yr findings of the FOCUS efficacy and safety study. Rheumatology (Oxford). 2009;48:188-194.
31. Perez-Ruiz F, Alonso-Ruiz A, Calabozo M, Herrero-Beites A, Garcia-Erauskin G, Ruiz-Lucea E. Efficacy of allopurinol and benzbromarone for the control of hyperuricaemia. A pathogenic approach to the treatment of primary chronic gout. Ann Rheum Dis. 1998;57:545-549.

32. Perez-Ruiz F, Calabozo M, Fernandez-Lopez MJ, et al. Treatment of chronic gout in patients with renal function impairment: an open, randomized, actively controlled study. *J Clin Rheumatol.* 1999;5:49-55.

33. Perez-Ruiz F, Gomez-Ullate P, Amenabar JJ, et al. Long-term efficacy of hyperuricaemia treatment in renal transplant patients. *Nephrol Dial Transplant.* 2003;18:603-606.

34. Pui K, Gow PJ, Dalbeth N. Efficacy and tolerability of probenecid as urate-lowering therapy in gout; clinical experience in high-prevalence. *J Rheumatol.* 2013;40:872-876.

35. Sundy JS, Hershfield MS. Uricase and other novel agents for the management of patients with treatment-failure gout. *Curr Rheum Rep.* 2007;9:258-264.

36. Edwards NL. Treatment-failure gout: a moving target. *Arthritis Rheum.* 2008;58:2587-2590.

37. Sherman MR, Saifer MGP, Perez-Ruiz F. PEG-uricase in the management of treatment-resistant gout and hyperuricemia. *Adv Drug Deliv Rev.* 2008;60:59-68.

38. European Medicines Agency Web site. Krystexxa Summary of Product Characteristics. http://www.ema.europa.eu/docs/en_GB/document_library/EPAR_-_Product_Information/human/002208/WC500138318.pdf. Accessed May 16, 2013.

39. Sundy JS, Baraf HSB, Yood RA, et al. Efficacy and tolerability of pegloticase for the treatment of chronic gout in patients refractory to conventional treatment: two randomized controlled trials. *JAMA.* 2011;306:711-720.

40. Perez-Ruiz F. New treatments for gout. *Bone Joint Spine.* 2007;74:313-315.

Chapter 5

Prevention and treatment of inflammation in gout

Fernando Perez-Ruiz and Alberto Alonso-Ruiz

Introduction

Acute inflammation is the hallmark of gout. Whereas episodes of acute inflammation (EAIs) are the paradigm of gout, chronic inflammation is related to the deposition of monosodium urate crystals (MSUCs) that is mostly subclinical and may appear early and even prior to the very first symptom [1]. This persistent, chronic inflammation can also occur during asymptomatic periods ('intercritical gout') [2]. Depletion of MSUCs is associated with a decrease both in EAIs and chronic inflammation; therefore, the aim of the treatment of gout is to completely and definitively deplete MSUCs from tissues.

Nevertheless, there is a certain, but transient risk of inducing EAIs when reducing serum urate levels (sUr) below the saturation threshold. This chapter will review the management of prevention of inflammation induced by MSUCs while starting urate-lowering therapy (ULT) and by treatment of intercurrent EAIs.

Local or national labels and recommendations should be carefully followed for all treatments discussed.

Prevention of episodes of acute inflammation in gout (prophylaxis)

Treatment to prevent EAIs has been associated with an improvement in patients´ reported outcomes, even in the absence of ULT

F. Perez-Ruiz and A. M. Herrero-Beites, *Managing Gout in Primary Care*, 53
DOI: 10.1007/978-1-907673-67-2_5, © Springer Healthcare 2014

implementation [3]. Although prevention of EAIs is a clinically desirable outcome for physicians and patients, the mere reduction in the number of EAIs should not be considered a target in itself, but a means to avoid patients' further suffering before MSUCs are dissolved and depleted from the tissues, and also to reduce healthcare resource utilization and costs that are intrinsically associated with the appearance of frequent EAIs [4].

When to start prophylaxis of EAIs

The recent 2012 guidelines of the American College of Rheumatology (ACR) state that "pharmacologic anti-inflammatory prophylaxis is recommended for all gout patients when pharmacologic urate lowering is initiated..." [5]. The ACR did not consider initiating prevention treatment for patients who start nonpharmacologic, effective ULT, such as lifestyle changes, or changes in medication that may be the cause of hyperuricemia (e.g., thiazide diuretics), as there are no trial data on which to base such a recommendation. The risk of inducing EAIs seems to be much higher when pharmacologic ULT is started, due to the rapidity and intensity in the reduction of sUr when urate-lowering medications (ULMs) are used [6].

It is common practice to start low-dose oral colchicine during the treatment of an EAI, if its use is not contraindicated. The ACR guidelines state that prevention treatment should be initiated with or just prior to initiating pharmacologic ULT [5,7].

How to achieve prophylaxis of EAIs

The sudden reduction of sUr is associated with an increase in the risk of EAIs, as observed in clinical trials in which patients were randomized to a high dose of febuxostat [8] or pegloticase [9]. Therefore, it is recommended that ULTs should be dosed with a step-up schedule [10]. A recent clinical trial showed that it made no difference whether allopurinol 300 mg/daily or placebo was prescribed to patients during an EAI, but considering that all patients received a full dose of colchicine (0.6 mg bid) for 90 days and high-dose indomethacin (50 mg tid) for the first 10 days [11], a limitation for the clinical applicability of these results is that combination of medications should only be prescribed to gouty but otherwise healthy patients. The reduction of serum urate observed with this dose of allopurinol is not comparable to the striking reduction of sUr that can be observed when potent ULMs such as benzbromarone, febuxostat, or pegloticase are used. In addition, a slow increase of allopurinol dosing is generally recommended due to safety concerns, especially in renally impaired patients [10].

The European League Against Rheumatism (EULAR) 2006 recommendations suggest that prevention against EAIs during the first months of ULT can be achieved with low-dose oral colchicine (0.5–1 mg/day) and/or non-steroidal anti-inflammatory drugs (NSAIDs), with gastroprotection if indicated [10]. The ACR guidelines note that low-dose oral colchicine and low-dose NSAIDs are both appropriate first-line prophylaxis therapy, unless not tolerated or contraindicated [5]. It should be noted that colchicine is not approved worldwide for the prevention of EAIs in gout, and neither are NSAIDs for asymptomatic patients, even at low doses.

Colchicine

Colchicine has been widely used for prevention of EAIs in clinical practice since the mid-20th century [12]. Its use is supported by two clinical trials [13,14], one using 0.5 mg tid and one using 0.6 mg bid orally, showing that at the oral dose two-thirds of the patients had mild adverse events. Colchicine for intravenous administration has been withdrawn in most countries due to serious safety concerns.

Colchicine is a lipophilic alkaloid with a high distribution volume (intracellular distribution) showing an apparent short half-life (rapid initial disappearance from plasma), but a long actual half-life that has to be carefully considered for prescription in clinical practice [14]. New evidence on its pharmacokinetics and interactions with other drugs [2] have increased the knowledge on how best to adapt prescriptions to the standards of efficacy and safety. Colchicine should be considered a drug with a narrow therapeutic margin for dosing.

Most anti-inflammatory effects of colchicine are likely due to disruption of microtubule function in activated neutrophils, which are pivotal in the generation of crystal-induced inflammation [15]. Approved doses for colchicine for the prevention of EAIs range from 0.5 to 0.6 mg once or twice daily. The pharmacokinetics of colchicine are altered in the presence of liver or kidney insufficiency, and this has meant that the previous recommendation supporting the idea that colchicine dose should be reduced in patients with kidney or liver dysfunction has been sustained [16].

Colchicine is metabolized by cytochrome P450 3A4 (CYP3A4) and is also a substrate for the P-glycoprotein transporter (or multidrug transporter-1). Therefore, pharmacokinetic interactions should be expected in patients taking medications that are strong inhibitors of CYP3A4 (including clarithromycin, telithromycin, ritonavir, ketoconazole, and itraconazole), strong inhibitors of the P-glycoprotein transporter (such as cyclosporine-A and tacrolimus), and moderate inhibitors of CYP3A4 (e.g., erythromycin, diltiazem, verapamil) [17,18]. It is recommended to reduce colchicine doses by 50% for patients who are also receiving moderate inhibitors of CYP3A4 or the P-glycoprotein transporter, and by 75% in patients on strong inhibitors [17]. Although it is not recommended to reduce the dose of colchicine in patients on medications that are mild inhibitors of CYP3A4 (such as statins), caution should be used or a further reduction of dose considered during follow-up of these patients, as colchicine has been shown to be associated with increased risk of adverse events [19], especially in the presence of renal or liver dysfunction [15].

When cautiously used, low-dose colchicine is usually well tolerated; the most frequent adverse events are abdominal cramps, soft stools, and diarrhea. Acute colchicine toxicity is manifested by severe gastrointestinal toxicity, bone marrow suppression, multiorgan failure, and even death. Chronic toxicity is most commonly expressed as neuromyopathy, with elevated creatine-kinase levels or bone marrow suppression [20].

Nonsteroidal anti-inflammatory drugs
In the EULAR guidelines, NSAIDs are recommended for the prevention of EAIs in patients intolerant of or contraindicated to colchicine or in countries where colchicine is not indicated [10]. The ACR also recommends low-dose NSAIDs (e.g., naproxen 250 mg bid) as first-line drugs for the prevention of EAIs [5]. Nevertheless, it has to be taken into consideration that this is an expert-based recommendation (grade C level of evidence), as no clinical trial has yet been published on the topic [5].

In addition, long-term chronic prescription of NSAIDs is not advisable for patients with clinically significant chronic kidney disease. In some countries, NSAID prescription is restricted to treat the signs and symptoms of inflammation, thus not including asymptomatic patients.

Corticosteroids

Low-dose corticosteroids (≤10 mg/day of equivalent prednisone) have been considered as alternatives for preventive treatment in patients with gout who show contraindications or in whom other medications may not be clinically acceptable [5]. It should be noted that in some countries, corticosteroids are approved only for symptomatic patients.

How long should prevention of EAIs be implemented?

The ACR guidelines state that "pharmacologic anti-inflammatory prophylaxis ... should be continued if there is any clinical evidence of continuing gout disease activity and/or the serum urate target has not yet been achieved" [5]. In addition, the ACR recommends maintaining prophylaxis in the absence of signs and symptoms of inflammation, for whichever time period is longer: at least 6 months (grade A level of recommendation); 3 months after proper control of sUr if no tophus is present in clinical examination (grade B level); or 6 months after proper control of sUr if any tophus is present in clinical examination (grade C level) [5].

Although data available to support these recommendations do not come directly from trials specifically designed to ascertain duration, short-term (2 months) treatment with colchicine or NSAIDs in the febuxostat trials was associated with a sudden increase in the incidence of EAIs (especially in patients on febuxostat 80–120 mg/day, who had the greatest decrease in sUr), whereas during a 6-month treatment period there was neither an increase in the number of EAIs nor an increase in adverse events [6].

Some indirect data may support longer duration of prophylaxis for patients with tophaceous gout; in one study <10% of patients without a tophus and who were not on prevention treatment suffered an EAI, whereas the incidence was 31% for patients with any tophus in clinical examination [7].

Treatment of episodes of acute inflammation in gout

Symptomatic relief of pain and inflammation is certainly an issue in clinical practice, especially in gout as it is thought to be the most painful cause of acute arthritis. Treating acute gout attacks alone is not sufficient to prevent the disease from progressing and should not jeopardize the final goal for the cure of gout, which is depleting MSUCs from tissues through the reduction of sUr levels.

Treatment of EAIs can be accomplished with different therapies, including physical measures and pharmacologic agents. The latter may include NSAIDs, colchicine, corticosteroids (administered either systemically or intra-articularly), and adrenocorticotropic hormone (ACTH) and its synthetic analogs (such as tetracosactide).

The key points for the success in treating EAIs are early treatment, choice of the drug to be prescribed based on the patient clinical profile (severity and extension of the EAI and the presence of comorbidities limiting certain drugs), and appropriate dosing to ascertain effectiveness and safety.

General measures

It is recommended to continue established pharmacologic ULT during an EAI [5], as withdrawal and/or initiation of ULT in the initial phase of treatment may be associated with increased risk of recurrences.

Different physical measures have been found to be useful as adjuvants to pharmacologic treatment to relieve pain and inflammation. Easing of the affected joints and resting them in such a position that reduces intra-articular pressure may alleviate the discomfort of the patient with gout and an EAI. Close splints or bandages are not recommended as they may compress the joint and increase pain through greater intra-articular pressure.

Careful, intermittent application of local ice packs has been shown to be useful in easing pain in patients with gout and other types of crystal-induced arthritis [21].

For a small number of patients who are intolerant to or contraindicated for all medications available, analgesics and physical measures may be the only method to minimize the pain until the inflammation spontaneously subsides.

Non-steroidal anti-inflammatory drugs

As noted earlier, NSAIDs are extremely effective at maximum labelled dosages to treat acute inflammation in gout and are the most commonly used medications in surveys [22] and research [23]. The EULAR Task Force has recommended that "in the absence of contraindications, an NSAID is a convenient and well accepted option" [10]. The ACR 2012 guidelines consider that NSAIDs, corticosteroids, or oral colchicine are appropriate first-line options for treatment of acute gout [5], as they have all shown to be highly effective.

There is scarce evidence from clinical trials that one NSAID may be more effective than another. The choice of NSAID may be based on the patient's and physician's previous experience, its availability, and especially its pharmacokinetics [24]. It should be noted that trials of NSAIDs in patients with gout have only included those with nonrefractory, non-polyarticular EAIs and no significant comorbid conditions and contraindications.

Colchicine

Early intake of low-dose colchicine may be an effective and safe treatment for EAIs of gout if it is not contraindicated. Colchicine has been widely used to successfully treat acute inflammation of gout for the last three centuries. Nevertheless, the risk of toxicity at doses commonly prescribed (up to 6 mg a day) is associated with a high rate of adverse events [25]. The EULAR recommendations included an expert-based commitment to use low-dose colchicine [10], but other experts have questioned whether there is still a place for colchicine in the gout treatment armamentarium [26].

A trial was designed to ascertain whether there was a difference in efficacy and safety between low-dose versus high-dose colchicine [27]. The results showed no difference in efficacy between arms but a significantly greater incidence of adverse events, mostly gastrointestinal, in the high-dose arm compared with lose-dose and placebo arms. This has led to changes in the label for colchicine in a number of countries. In addition, in the above trial, colchicine was self-administered once the patient felt the initiation of an EAI. Thus, some experts consider that colchicine should be considered an 'in-the-pocket medication,' prescribed in advance and to be used as soon as the patient is sure that an EAI is developing [28]. Patients' perception of having a flare is validated when it is supported by self-perceived presence of pain and joint swelling [29].

One limitation to the advanced prescription of colchicine for the treatment of EAIs would be when colchicine is used for the prevention of EAIs; in such cases the patient would already be on low-dose colchicine and so there will be a limited potential for further dose increases (according to maximum labelled doses). Therefore, in these situations, the ACR guidelines suggest using alternative treatments, such as NSAIDs or corticosteroids [5]. Another consideration is that there are currently no published head-to-head trial data comparing the efficacy and safety of colchicine with NSAIDs or corticosteroids to treat EAIs of gout.

Corticosteroids

Corticosteroids are highly effective in controlling the signs and symptoms of acute inflammation of gout. The ACR guidelines recommend doses of 0.5 mg/kg/day of prednisone equivalent [5].

Systemic corticosteroids

Trials comparing NSAIDs and corticosteroids have shown no difference between therapies [30,31]. This was also shown in a recent systematic review comparing corticosteroids to NSAIDs [32], but it was based only on three trials with poor quality of design. Furthermore, patients had nonsevere EAIs and no comorbidities, and most of them showed monoarticular and early presentation, with involvement of the first metatarsophalangeal joint of the feet only [33]. Another trial compared indomethacin/paracetamol with paracetamol/prednisone, although patients in the indomethacin arm were in fact pre-treated with intramuscular diclofenac, thus receiving two NSAIDs, a practice not widely accepted by regulatory agencies [31].

Corticosteroids may be considered as an alternative treatment in patients with contraindications to NSAIDs and colchicine, or in whom these drugs are not clinically appropriate [10]. Limitations for their use include presence or suspicion of infection, either local or at other locations, and concomitant diabetes.

The risk of abuse associated with corticosteroids may favor extended tophaceous deposition in patients abusing and not taking the medication as prescribed or showing no urate-lowering effectiveness [34]. There is therefore some debate about whether oral or parenteral corticosteroids should be administered at all, in order to avoid this risk [10].

Intra-articular corticosteroids

Intra-articular injection of corticosteroids also seemed to be effective in open-label studies [35]. Limitations for administering intra-articular corticosteroids include skills for puncturing and aspirating joints (culture of synovial fluid is advisable if obtained), a reasonable certainty that the patient does not have ongoing infectious arthritis, and the need for onsite availability of a physician with experience in administering these drugs.

Articular injection of corticosteroids could also be considered for patients with a single, accessible joint affected during the EAI, as aspirating and injecting multiple joints does not make sense for clinical practice [5].

ACTH and its analogs

ACTH was first used to treat EAIs of gout over 50 years ago [36], but its actual mechanism was not discovered until recently [37]. The drug and its approved analogs, such as tetracosactide, share a common mechanism of inducing the activation of neutrophil melanocortin receptor 3, which exerts an anti-inflammatory effect. The efficacy of parenteral administration of ACTH is similar to that of oral indomethacin [38]. This mechanism of action seems to be an attractive one for further clinical investigation [39]. The only registered clinical trial of ACTH is currently ongoing in the EU. A recent retrospective review of nearly two hundred patients showed a high rate of effectiveness of ACTH in controlling acute inflammation of gout, with a favorable safety profile even in patients with diabetes [40].

Limitations of ACTH use is its short half-life that may necessitate repeated administration, although a depot preparation of tetracosactide is available in some European countries. There is a lack of randomized, double-blind clinical trials data as well as prospective evaluations of safety, especially when repeated injections are prescribed [39].

Combination treatment

Reports from a published survey indicate that in the US, a combination of different medications is often used to treat EAIs [22]. The ACR 2012 guidelines suggest that certain combinations of medications can be employed for severe or refractory attacks if the individual agents are not contraindicated [5]. Combination treatment may be initially considered as appropriate management for severe EAIs, defined as those involving several large joints or multiple joints. In addition, patients with no response to a single medication can also be considered for combination treatment after diagnostic re-evaluation [5].

The combination approaches considered as acceptable by the ACR experts include the simultaneous administration of oral colchicine (full doses or, where appropriate, prophylaxis doses) and NSAIDs, oral colchicine and oral corticosteroids, and intra-articular injection of corticosteroids plus oral administration of any of the other medications. No recommendation is available for the combination of corticosteroids and NSAIDs [5].

Emerging approaches: interleukin-1 antagonists

As described in Chapter 2, interleukin-1 (IL-1) is thought to be a major effector of the inflammatory response induced by MSUCs through the sequential activation of the inflammasome NALP3 and caspase-1. Canakinumab, a human monoclonal antibody approved for use against IL-1β, has been recently given an extension of label by the European Medicines Agency (EMA) for the treatment of the EAIs of gout under restricted circumstances: at least three EAIs a year; contraindication for both NSAIDs and colchicine; and when repeated treatment with systemic corticosteroids is not clinically acceptable.

Other IL-1 antagonists not approved for use in gout include anakinra (an antagonist of the IL-1 receptor, approved for juvenile arthritis) and rilonacept (an IL-1 trap, approved for the treatment of cryopirin-associated syndromes) [41].

The effectiveness of the blockade of IL-1 to treat EAIs of gout was first demonstrated using anakinra in an open, non-comparative study [42], but no data from randomized controlled trials have been released. Rilonacept has been shown to be useful for prevention of the EAIs of gout at the start of ULM therapy [43,44], but failed to demonstrate further benefit when added to indomethacin to treat EAIs [45]. Canakinumab was more effective than parenteral triamcinolone at single doses, and canakinumab administration was also associated with lower risk of recurrence [46,47].

The limitation of IL-1 antagonists are that only canakinumab has been approved for the treatment of EAIs of gout, none are approved for prevention of EAIs, and their use is associated with an increased risk of infections.

Key points

- Prevention of EAIs is recommended when starting ULT.
- Prophylaxis should be continued for 3 to 6 months after symptoms have definitively subsided, depending on the situation.
- Low-dose colchicine, low-dose NSAIDs, and low-dose corticosteroids may be considered, depending on the clinical situation and national labels and recommendations where available.
- Early treatment of the EAIs of gout will improve response to medications.
- A combination of medications may be considered initially for patients with severe EAIs or subsequently in patients with insufficient response to monotherapy.
- IL-1 antagonists are promising medications for the prevention and treatment of urate crystal-induced inflammation.

References

1 De Miguel E, Puig JG, Castillo C, Peiteado D, Torres RJ, Martín-Mola E. Diagnosis of gout in patients with asymptomatic hyperuricemia: a pilot ultrasound study. *Ann Rheum Dis*. 2011;71:157-158.

2 Wright SA, Filippucci E, McVeigh C, et al. High resolution ultrasonography of the first metatarsal phalangeal joint in gout: a controlled study. *Ann Rheum Dis*. 2007;66:859-864.

3 Khanna PP, Perez-Ruiz F, Maranian P, Khanna D. Long-term therapy for chronic gout results in clinically important improvements in the health-related quality of life: short form-36 is responsive to change in chronic gout. *Rheumatology (Oxford)*. 2011;50:740-745.

4 Saseen JJ, Agashivala N, Allen RR, Ghushchyan V, Yadao AM, Nair KV. Comparison of patient characteristics and gout-related health-care resource utilization and costs in patients with frequent versus infrequent gouty arthritis attacks. *Rheumatology (Oxford)*. 2012;51: 2004-2012.

5 Khanna D, Khanna PP, Fitzgerald JD, et al. 2012 American College of Rheumatology guidelines for management of gout. Part 2: Therapy and antiinflammatory prophylaxis of acute gouty arthritis. *Arthritis Care Res (Hoboken)*. 2012;64:1447-1461.

6 Wortmann RL, MacDonald PA, Hunt B, Jackson RL. Effect of prophylaxis on gout flares after the initiation of urate-lowering therapy: analysis of data from three Phase III trials. *Clin Ther*. 2010;32:2386-2397.

7 Schumacher HR Jr, Becker MA, Lloyd E, MacDonald PA, Lademacher C. Febuxostat in the treatment of gout: 5-yr findings of the FOCUS efficacy and safety study. *Rheumatology*. 2009;48:188-194.

8 Becker MA, Schumacher HR Jr, Wortmann RL, et al. Febuxostat compared with allopurinol in patients with hyperuricemia and gout. *N Engl J Med*. 2005;353:2450-2461.

9 Sundy JS, Baraf HSB, Yood RA, et al. Efficacy and tolerability of pegloticase for the treatment of chronic gout in patients refractory to conventional treatment: two randomized controlled trials. *JAMA*. 2011;306:711-720.

10 Zhang W, Doherty M, Bardin T, et al. EULAR evidence based recommendations for gout. Part II. Management. Report of a Task Force of the EULAR Standing Committee for international clinical studies including therapeutics (ESCISIT). *Ann Rheum Dis*. 2006;65:1312-1324.

11 Taylor TH, Mecchella JN, Larson RJ, Kerin KD, Mackenzie TA. Initiation of allopurinol at first medical contact for acute attacks of gout: a randomized clinical trial. *Am J Med*. 2012;125:1126-1134.

12 Yü TF, Gutman AB. Efficacy of colchicine prophylaxis in gout: prevention of recurrent gouty arthritis over a mean period of five years in 208 gouty subjects. *Ann Intern Med*. 1961;55: 179-192.

13 Paulus HE, Schlosstein LH, Godfrey RG, Klinenberg JR, Bluestone R. Prophylactic colchicine therapy of intercritical gout: a placebo-controlled study of probenecid-treated patients. *Arthritis Rheum*. 1974;17:609-614.

14 Borstad GC, Bryant LR, Abel MP, Scroggie DA, Harris MD, Alloway JA. Colchicine for prophylaxis of acute flares when initiating allopurinol for chronic gouty arthritis. *J Rheumatol*. 2004;31:2429-2432.

15 Terkeltaub RA. Colchicine update: 2008. Semin Arthritis Rheum. 2009;38:411-419.

16 Yang LPH. Oral colchicine (Colcrys®) in the treatment and prophylaxis of gout. *Drugs*. 2010;70:1603-1613.

17 Terkeltaub RA, Furst DE, DiGiacinto JL, Kook KA, Davis MW. Novel evidence-based colchicine dose-reduction algorithm to predict and prevent colchicine toxicity in the presence of cytochrome P450 3A4/P-glycoprotein inhibitors. *Arthritis Rheum*. 2011;63:2226-2237.

18 Davis MW, Wason S, DiGiacinto JL. Colchicine-antimicrobial drug interactions: what pharmacists need to know in treating gout. *Consult Pharm*. 2013;28:176-183.

19 Ryu HJ, Song R, Kim HW, et al. Clinical risk factors for adverse events in allopurinol users [published online ahead of print January 24, 2013]. *J Clin Pharmacol*. doi: 10.1177/0091270011439715.

20 Kuncl RW, Duncan G, Watson , Alderson K, Rogawsky MA, Peper M. Colchicine miopathy and neuropathy. *N Engl J Med*. 1987;25:1552-1568.

21 Schlesinger N. Response to application of ice may help differentiate between gouty arthritis and other inflammatory arthritides. *J Clin Rheumatol*. 2006;12:275-276.

22 Schlesinger N, Moore DF, Sun JD, Schumacher HR Jr. A survey of current evaluation and treatment of gout. *J Rheumatol*. 2006;33:2050-2052.

23 Perez-Ruiz F, Carmona L, Yebeñes MJG, et al; on behalf of the GEMA Study Group, Sociedad Española de Reumatología. An audit of the variability of diagnosis and management of gout in the rheumatology setting: the Gout Evaluation and Management study. *J Clin Rheumatol*. 2011;17:349-355.

24 Perez-Ruiz F, Gonzalez Mielgo FJ, Herrero-Beites AM. Optimisation of the treatment of acute gout. *BioDrugs*. 2000;13:45-53.

25 Ahern MJ, Reid C, Gordon TP, McCredie M, Brooks PM, Jones M. Does colchicine work? The results of the first controlled study in acute gout. *Aust NZ J Med*. 1987;17:301-304.

26 Grahame R. Is there still a place for colchicine in the treatment of acute gout? *Int J Clin Pract*. 2007;61:1966-1967.

27 Terkeltaub RA, Furst DE, Bennett K, Kook KA, Crockett RS, Davis MW. High versus low dosing of oral colchicine for early acute gout flare: twenty-four-hour outcome of the first multicenter, randomized, double-blind, placebo-controlled, parallel-group, dose-comparison colchicine study. *Arthritis Rheum*. 2010;62:1060-1068.

28 Richette P, Bardin T. Colchicine for the treatment of gout. *Expert Opin Pharmacother*. 2010;11:2933-2938.

29 Gaffo AL, Schumacher HR, Saag KG, et al. Developing a provisional definition of flare in patients with established gout. *Arthritis Rheum*. 2012;64:1508-1517.

30 Alloway JA, Moriarty MJ, Hoogland YT, Nashel DJ. Comparison of triamcinolone acetonide with indomethacin in the treatment of acute gouty arthritis. *J Rheumatol*. 1993;20:111-113.

31 Man CY, Cheung ITF, Cameron PA, Rainer TH. Comparison of oral prednisolone/paracetamol and oral indomethacin/paracetamol combination therapy in the treatment of acute goutlike arthritis: a double-blind, randomized, controlled trial. *Ann Emerg Med*. 2007;49:670-677.

32 Janssens HJ, Lucassen PLBJ, Van de Laar FA, Janssen M, Van de Lisdonk EH. Systemic corticosteroids for acute gout. *Cochrane Database Syst Rev*. 2008:CD005521.

33 Janssens HJEM, Janssen M, van de Lisdonk EH, van Riel PLCM, van Weel C. Use of oral prednisolone or naproxen for the treatment of gout arthritis: a double-blind, randomised equivalence trial. Lancet. 2008;371:1854-1860.

34 Vázquez-Mellado J, Cuan A, Magaña M, et al. Intradermal tophi in gout: a case-control study. *J Rheumatol*. 1999;26:136-140.

35 Fernández C, Noguera R, González JA, Pascual E. Treatment of acute attacks of gout with a small dose of intraarticular triamcinolone acetonide. J Rheumatol. 1999;26:2285-2286.

36 Gutman AB, Yü TF. Effects of adrenocorticotropic hormone (ACTH) in gout. *Am J Med*. 1950;9:24-30.

37 Getting SJ, Christian HC, Flower RJ, Perretti M. Activation of melanocortin type 3 receptor as a molecular mechanism for adrenocorticotropic hormone efficacy in gouty arthritis. *Arthritis Rheum*. 2002;46:2765-2775.

38 Axelrod D, Preston S. Comparison of parenteral adrenocorticotropic hormone with oral indomethacin in the treatment of acute gout. *Arthritis Rheum*. 1988;31:803-805.

39 Perez-Ruiz F, Herrero-Beites AM. ACTH analogues medications for the treatment of crystal-induced acute inflammation. A target to be explored? [published online ahead of print March 19, 2013] *Joint Bone Spine*. doi: 10.1016/j.jbspin.2013.01.009.

40 Daoussis D, Antonopoulos I, Yiannopoulos G, Andonopoulos AP. ACTH as first line treatment for acute gout in 181 hospitalized patients. Joint Bone Spine. 2013;80:291-294.

41 So A, Busso N. A magic bullet for gout? *Ann Rheum Dis*. 2009;68;1517-1519.

42 So A, De Smedt T, Revaz S, Tschopp J. A pilot study of IL-1 inhibition by anakinra in acute gout. *Arthritis Res Ther*. 2007;9:R28.

43 Mitha E, Schumacher HR, Fouche L, et al. Rilonacept for gout flare prevention during initiation of uric acid-lowering therapy: results from the PRESURGE-2 international, phase 3, randomized, placebo-controlled trial [published online ahead of print March 13, 2013]. *Rheumatology (Oxford)*. doi: 10.1093/rheumatology/ket114.

44 Schumacher HR Jr, Evans RR, Saag KG, et al. Rilonacept (Interleukin-1 Trap) for prevention of gout flares during initiation of uric acid-lowering therapy: Results of the presurge-1 trial. *Arthritis Care Res (Hoboken)*. 2012;64:1462-1470.

45 Terkeltaub RA, Schumacher HR, Carter JD, et al. Rilonacept in the treatment of acute gouty arthritis: a randomized, controlled clinical trial using indomethacin as the active comparator. *Arthritis Res Ther*. 2013;15:R25.

46 Schlesinger N, Schumacher HR, Bardin T, et al. Efficacy of canakinumab versus triamcinolone acetonide in acute gouty arthritis patients: results of the B-Relieved II study (response in acute flare and in prevention of episodes of re-flare in gout). *Ann Rheum Dis*. 2011;70(suppl 3):186. Abstract THU0019.

47 So A, Alten R, Bardin T, et al. A controlled trial of canakinumab vs triamcinolone acetonide in acute gouty arthritis patients: results of the B-Relieved study (response in acute flare and in prevention of episodes of re-flare in gout). *Ann Rheum Dis*. 2011;70(suppl 3):104. Abstract OP0108.

Appendix

Summary of the 2006 European League Against Rheumatism (EULAR)
Task Force for Gout Recommendations and the 2012 American
College of Rheumatology (ACR) Guidelines for Management of Gout
Ana-María Herrero Beites and Fernando Perez Ruiz

General approach: lifestyle recommendations, education, and comorbid conditions

EULAR [1]
- Optimal treatment of gout requires both nonpharmacologic and pharmacologic modalities.
- Associated comorbidity and risk factors such as hyperlipidemia, hypertension, hyperglycemia, obesity, and smoking should be addressed as an important part of the management of gout.
- Patient education and appropriate lifestyle advice regarding weight loss if obese, diet, and reduced alcohol intake (especially beer) are core aspects of management.
- When gout is associated with diuretic therapy, stop the diuretic if possible; for hypertension and hyperlipidemia treatment, consider the use of losartan and fenofibrate, respectively.

ACR [2]
- Patient education on diet, lifestyle, treatment objectives, and management of comorbidities is a recommended core therapeutic measure in gout.

Diagnosis, evaluation of severity of disease, and suggestions for referral comment

EULAR [3]
- Demonstration of monosodium urate crystals (MSUCs) in synovial fluid or tophus aspirates permits a definitive diagnosis of gout.
- Identification of MSUCs from asymptomatic joints may allow definite diagnosis in intercritical periods.
- A routine search for MSUCs is recommended in all synovial fluid samples obtained from undiagnosed inflamed joints.
- Gout and sepsis may coexist, so when septic arthritis is suspected, Gram stain and culture of synovial fluid should still be performed even if MSUCs are identified.
- While high sUr levels is the most important risk factor for gout, they do not confirm or exclude gout as many people with hyperuricemia do not develop gout, and during acute attacks sUr may be normal.
- For typical presentations of gout (such as recurrent podagra with hyperuricemia), a clinical diagnosis alone is reasonably accurate but not definitive without crystal confirmation.

F. Perez-Ruiz and A. M. Herrero-Beites, *Managing Gout in Primary Care*, 67
DOI: 10.1007/978-1-907673-67-2, © Springer Healthcare 2014

- In acute attacks, the rapid development of severe pain, swelling, and tenderness that reaches its maximum within 6–12 hours, especially with overlying erythema, is highly suggestive of crystal inflammation, though is not specific for gout.
- Although radiographs may be useful for differential diagnosis and may show typical features in chronic gout, they are not useful in confirming the diagnosis of early or acute gout.
- Renal uric acid excretion should be determined in certain patients with gout, especially those with a family history of early-onset gout, onset of gout under age 25, or renal calculi.
- Risk factors for gout and associated comorbidities should be assessed, including features of the metabolic syndrome (obesity, hyperglycemia, hyperlipidemia, and hypertension).

ACR [4]

- Clinically evaluate gout disease burden: palpable tophi and severity of acute and chronic signs and symptoms.
- Gout case scenarios where referral to a specialist is considered include:
  - Unclear etiology of hyperuricemia.
  - Refractory signs and symptoms of gout.
  - Difficulty in reaching sUr target, particularly with renal impairment and a trial of XOI treatment.
  - Multiple and/or serious adverse events caused by pharmacologic ULT.

Urate-lowering therapy

EULAR [1]

- Urate-lowering therapy (ULT) is indicated in patients with recurrent acute attacks, arthropathy, tophi, or radiographic changes of gout.
- The therapeutic goal of ULT is to promote crystal dissolution and prevent crystal formation; this is achieved by maintaining the serum uric acid below the saturation point for monosodium urate (6 mg/dL or 360 µmol/L).
- Allopurinol is an appropriate long-term urate-lowering drug; it should be started at a low dose and increased by 100 mg every 2–4 weeks if required.
- If allopurinol toxicity occurs, treatment options include other xanthine oxidase inhibitors (XOIs) or a uricosuric agent.
- Uricosuric agents can be used as an alternative to allopurinol in patients without urolithiasis.

ACR [4]

- Pharmacologic ULT is indicated in patients with established diagnosis of gouty arthritis and:
  - Tophus or tophi by clinical exam or imaging study
  - Frequent attacks of gouty arthritis (>1/ year)
  - Chronic kidney disease (CKD) stage 2 or worse (estimated clearance of creatinine <90 mL/min)
  - Past urolithiasis
- Consider elimination of nonessential prescription of medications that induce hyperuricemia.
- XOI therapy with either allopurinol or febuxostat is recommended as the first-line pharmacologic ULT approach in gout.
- The starting dose of allopurinol should be ≤100 mg/day and less than that in moderate-to-severe chronic kidney disease, followed by gradual upward titration of the maintenance dose, which can exceed 300 mg/day even in patients with CKD.
- Serum urate (sUr) level should be lowered sufficiently to durably improve signs and symptoms of gout, with a target of 6 mg/dL (360 µmol/L) at a minimum, and often 5 mg/dL (300 µmol/L) (for patients with severe disease).
- After palpable tophi and all acute and chronic arthritis gout symptoms have resolved, continue all measures, including pharmacologic ULT, needed to maintain sUr level <6 mg/dL (360 µmol/L).
- The combination of an oral ULT with one XOI agent and one uricosuric agent is appropriate when the sUr target has not been met by appropriate dosing of an XOI.

- Pegloticase is appropriate for patients with severe gout disease burden and refractoriness to, or intolerance of, appropriately dosed oral ULT options.

Prevention of episodes of acute inflammation

EULAR [1]
- Prophylaxis against acute attacks during the first months of ULT can be achieved by colchicine (0.5–1 mg daily) and/or a non-steroidal anti-inflammatory drug (NSAID) (with gastroprotection if indicated)

ACR [4]
- Pharmacologic anti-inflammatory prophylaxis is recommended for all patients with gout when pharmacologic urate lowering is initiated, and should be continued if there is any clinical evidence of continuing gout disease activity and/or the serum urate target has not yet been achieved.
- Oral colchicine is an appropriate first-line prophylaxis therapy for episodes of acute inflammation (EAIs) of gout, with appropriate dose adjustment for CKD and drug interactions, unless there is a lack of tolerance or medical contraindication.
- Low-dose NSAID therapy is an appropriate choice for first-line gout attack prophylaxis, unless there is a lack of tolerance or medical contraindication.
- Prophylaxis should last the greater of: at least 6 months; 3 months after proper control of sUr levels if no tophus is present in clinical examination; or 6 months after proper control of sUr if any tophus is present in clinical examination (grade of level of recommendation C).

Treatment of the episodes of acute inflammation

EULAR [1]
- Oral colchicine and/or NSAIDs are first-line agents for systemic treatment of acute attacks; in the absence of contraindications, an NSAID is a convenient and well-accepted option.
- High doses of colchicine lead to side effects, and low doses may be sufficient for some patients with acute gout.
- Intra-articular aspiration and injection of a long-acting corticosteroid is an effective and safe treatment for an acute attack.

ACR [4]
- An EAI of gout should be treated with pharmacologic therapy, initiated within 24 hours of onset.
- Established pharmacologic ULT should be continued, without interruption, during an EAI of gout.
- NSAIDs, corticosteroids, or oral colchicine are appropriate first-line options for treatment of acute gout, and certain combinations can be employed for severe or refractory attacks.

References

1. Zhang W, Doherty M, Bardin T, et al. EULAR evidence based recommendations for gout. Part II. Management. Report of a task force of the EULAR Standing Committee for International Clinical Studies Including Therapeutics (ESCISIT). *Ann Rheum Dis*. 2006;65:1312-1324.
2. Khanna D, Fitzgerald JD, Khanna PP, et al. 2012 American College of Rheumatology guidelines for management of gout. Part 1: Systematic nonpharmacologic and pharmacologic therapeutic approaches to hyperuricemia. *Arthritis Care Res (Hoboken)*. 2012;64:1431-1446.
3. Zhang W, Doherty M, Pascual E, et al. EULAR evidence based recommendations for gout, Part I. Diagnosis. Report of a task force of the EULAR Standing,Committee for International Clinical Studies Including Therapeutics (ESCISIT). *Ann Rheum Dis*. 2006;65:1301-1311.
4. Khanna D, Khanna PP, Fitzgerald JD, et al. 2012 American College of Rheumatology guidelines for management of gout. Part 2: Therapy and antiinflammatory prophylaxis of acute gouty arthritis. *Arthritis Care Res (Hoboken)*. 2012;64:1447-1461.